Responses to a Pandemic

Responses to a Pandemic

Philosophical and Political Reflections

Edited by Anna Gotlib

ROWMAN & LITTLEFIELD
Lanham • Boulder • New York • London

Published by Rowman & Littlefield
An imprint of The Rowman & Littlefield Publishing Group, Inc.
4501 Forbes Boulevard, Suite 200, Lanham, Maryland 20706
www.rowman.com

86-90 Paul Street, London EC2A 4NE

British Library Cataloguing in Publication Information Available

Library of Congress Cataloging-in-Publication Data

Names: Gotlib, Anna, editor.
Title: Responses to a pandemic : philosophical and political reflections / edited by Anna Gotlib.
Description: [Lanham, MD] : [Rowman & Littlefield Publishers], [2022] | Includes bibliographical references and index.
Identifiers: LCCN 2022025835 (print) | LCCN 2022025836 (ebook) | ISBN 9781538154045 (cloth) | ISBN 9781538154069 (paperback) | ISBN 9781538154052 (epub)
Subjects: LCSH: COVID-19 Pandemic, 2020--Philosophy. | COVID-19 Pandemic, 2020--Political aspects. | COVID-19 Pandemic, 2020--Social aspects. | COVID-19 (Disease)
Classification: LCC RA644.C67 R467 2022 (print) | LCC RA644.C67 (ebook) | DDC 362.1962/414–dc23/eng/20220713
LC record available at https://lccn.loc.gov/2022025835
LC ebook record available at https://lccn.loc.gov/2022025836

For Jay. And for all those lost to the pandemic.

Contents

Acknowledgments

So much of life prior to March 2020 seems distant, submerged in a semi-nostalgic fog for the "before times." Now, with more than seven hundred thousand deaths in the United States and more than 4.8 million worldwide, we find ourselves in a different place—physically, psychologically, politically, morally. But as we try to adjust to whatever is "the new normal," we wonder what normal might be anymore. And we are haunted by what was, by *who* was, by who is no longer. While we who are left somehow persist, we persist in a grief-haunted world.

This book is the result of this sense of being haunted. As a philosopher who writes about, among other things, negative emotions such as sadness, regret, nostalgia, and the experiences of trauma, my first impulse was to examine what this sense is like—not abstractly, not hypothetically, not "for people in general," but for individuals who just happen to be philosophers. I asked my contributors: What is it that the last almost two years have done to you, to those you love, to your profession, to your sense of the world? What do you want to say to all those out there who do not necessarily share a philosopher's preoccupation with discipline-specific discourses—how would you talk to others who might want to hear you as simply one person to another? In doing so, I was thinking about "Diving into the Wreck," wherein the poet Adrienne Rich tells us of "the thing I came for:/the wreck and not the story of the wreck/the thing itself and not the myth."[1] The essays found in this volume, I believe, offer stories, yes—but stories that reveal rather than obfuscate. Importantly, they communicate many versions of the "thing itself" as found by each writer, struggling through the wreckage of the pandemic.

This book is also the result of my own prolonged, perhaps shocked, silence. Shortly before COVID-19 was recognized as a worldwide pandemic and so many of us retreated into our homes, I returned from a Fulbright Specialist fellowship, having taught at the University of Iceland in the early part of the winter semester in 2020. As my partner and I were making our way through Keflavík airport, we kept noticing the relative lack of travelers, the mask-wearing employees, the hand sanitizer, the tension. Upon landing at JFK, while the chaos and the general overcrowding were as expected, among those waiting to be screened back into the city, I began to hear about "a really bad flu," "something contagious," or "something pretty bad happening in China." Having noted the growing attention to this strange new virus in the increasingly alarmed media, I began to worry, my bioethics training kicking in: Is this "the one"?

It was. And for quite some time, all I could do was try to take in what was going on all around us: the lockdowns and stay-at-home orders, the injustices felt by "essential workers" who had no such luxury, the heroic medical staff, the political demagoguery, the deaths, the fear. My God, the fear. As a philosopher—as a *person*—I was out of reasons, out of words, out of explanations. In the sudden switch to online teaching, I saw the bewildered, frightened faces of my students, some of whom lived in the very worst, most pandemic-stricken parts of the city. Staring at each other through strange, unfamiliar boxes on a screen, we all tried to make sense of a syllabus, of a course that only a few weeks ago seemed so sensibly and effectively put together—indeed, of a world where we read about doctor-patient relationships at the exact moment these relationships were reaching their breaking point at a hospital down the block. And as I tried to hold them together, I tried to also hold myself together. Sometimes, that meant admitting that neither was possible.

As the pandemic became more and more of a constant with no end in sight, it occurred to me that we, as philosophers, ought to start speaking. So I began slowly, by writing pieces about COVID-19 and anxiety; about what "optimism" might mean now, in its grip; about how to understand trauma as something other than an end to everything. But it also became clear that more needed to be said—and not just to other philosophers. For weeks, this odd idea of a "philosophers' pandemic diary" kept running through my mind, but no substantive ideas about how to frame it came. Then one day, in a moment of uncharacteristic impulsivity, I issued a call for papers for a volume on philosophical reflections on COVID-19 aimed at the general public. Almost immediately, my colleagues replied: enthusiastically, generously, creatively. This volume is their response, and thus my primary gratitude is to them: to all those who contributed their wonderful, personal narratives; to all those who wanted to do so, but because of what the pandemic has made of us all, could not; to all those who encouraged me along the way. Thank you, from the bottom of my heart. I am also, and always, grateful to my friend, mentor, and true north—Hilde Lindemann—for the encouragement, for the confidence. For the love. Thank you as well to my wonderful colleagues in the philosophy department at Brooklyn College for always supporting, and never judging, the weird projects in which I tend to engage. I am also grateful to my editors and staff at Rowman & Littlefield International for their initial enthusiasm for the project, as well as for the support along the way. Of course, I will always be grateful to my students, who never fail to remind me how necessary it is that philosophers and other academics talk *with*, and not *at*, all those who may not be familiar with our strange insider discourses. And finally, I will be forever and always grateful to my best friend, my constant support system, and my love—my partner, Jeff Guevin. Nothing would be possible without you—ever.

One concluding acknowledgment: As the pandemic was beginning its deadly march around the world, we New Yorkers, at least for a while, continued to go on as usual: we went to work, we met in large groups, we took the subway. Until many of us didn't. For me, March 10, 2020, was the last day I saw my office in Brooklyn College, the last day my colleagues and I exchanged worried, anxious glances while in a single room together. And it was the last day that I would see Jay Jankelewicz, our wonderful philosophy department office manager, alive. Jay was one of COVID-19's earlier victims, succumbing to the virus in April 2020, just as New York City began to feel its first brutal grip. This book is dedicated to Jay—our irrepressible, irreplaceable, wonderful Jay—and to all those others who perished in the tragedy to which we, *in medias res*, are bearing witness. It is my sincerest hope that we bear it well, together.

NOTE

1. Adrienne Rich, *Diving into the Wreck: Poems, 1971–1972* (New York: Norton, 1973).

In Medias Res: Philosophers as Witnesses to Disaster

Anna Gotlib

INTRODUCTION

Unlike many philosophical efforts, this volume is neither a response to an ongoing scholarly debate, nor the result of rarefied research, nor a circumscribed contribution to perceived gaps in academic literature. Instead, it is an attempt at broad public engagement born of a desire to communicate the shared human ordeals of pandemic anxieties, fears, frustrations, and traumas in ways that are immediate, visceral, and, I believe, necessary. This multivocal and diverse collection adds philosophers' voices to the challenges of facing, naming, and examining what this now two-year-long juggernaut of COVID-19 has done to us—to *all* of us—and how we might begin to make sense of our experiences. And to talk back to them.

This book is unusual in other respects, as well. A collection of responses by philosophers to the current pandemic, it is neither a strictly philosophical debate intended for insiders, nor an introductory text for beginners. It is instead an extended narrative of the many phenomenologies of this pandemic: it is about reactions to, and personal stories of, our pain, fear, challenges, and anxieties; it is about the pandemic's revelatory effects on us individually and as a society; it is about the changes it has wrought upon the world as we know it. In short, it is a book of narratives about personal experiences in the midst of a pandemic by people who happen to be philosophers, rather than a philosophical debate, or an analysis of the pandemic, through an academic lens.

Because I am a philosopher and a bioethicist by training, my decision to limit the contributors in this volume to other academics is perhaps not surprising—and, I hope, not disappointing. While the contributions are not only personal, but moving, insightful, and illuminating, there is an additional reason for my selections. Turning to philosophers for this volume had less to do with a preference for certain kinds of scholars, or for certain perspectives on this very public, very global disaster, and more to do with the fact that philosophy as a discipline, at least in my view, is in the middle of two fundamental transitions. First, in shifting from largely abstract, and somewhat limited, focus on questions deemed to be sufficiently "philosophical," philosophy is (slowly and imperfectly) expanding its universe to include the kinds of questions that do not center specialized jargon or technical obscurantism, instead focusing on the actual lived lives of persons. Second, somewhat freed from the shackles of worries about whether one's project was properly "philosophical," some scholars have increasingly begun to address audiences who were neither philosophers nor professional academics—and what is known as "public philosophy" has gained not only adherents among its practitioners, but increasing interest among more general readers. This volume is offered in the spirit of expanding the scope of philosophical engagement in general, and of the public philosophy movement in particular.

IN MEDIAS RES

Perhaps too much of academic, and especially philosophical, writing takes place after the fact. In moral philosophy, ethical dilemmas are analyzed (mostly) long after the actual events in question; in bioethics, case studies are examined as a way of looking at the past to better understand how to proceed with current and future decisions; in political philosophy, theorists reflect on historical events to help conceptualize the ones before us now. And although I am quite certain that libraries will be filled with books dedicated to examining the big biomedical, moral, political, and social questions raised by the current pandemic, this is not my intent here. Instead, this volume attempts to consider our current global disaster from the inside, by the same people who must navigate their personal and professional realities while in the middle of the pandemic. This *in medias res* perspective is not only challenging personally for the writer—opening oneself up, especially after over two years of ongoing trauma, always is—but also asks much of the reader: it asks for understanding, for empathy, for patience, for a generosity to the often-unfamiliar inner worlds of others in ways that philosophy too often ignores. If successful, perhaps the reader can see herself a bit more clearly through the writer; perhaps the writer can see herself a bit more clearly in her attempt to make that connection happen. And this *matters*— after all, it seems to me that in isolation, we, as human beings, have never been that good at seeing ourselves.

In deciding to put this collection together, I had to do a bit of negotiating with myself as someone who is generally wary of writing (or asking others to write) without at least some minimal distance from the topic at hand. What finally motivated me to cease negotiations and proceed was the urgency of our (unequally) shared suffering, the seeming intractability of our challenges, and the depth of our despair. I say "our" because in the era of COVID-19, there is very little distinction between academia and everyone else: nobody is completely removed from the pandemic—although, as a number of contributors point out, certain individuals and groups are much better protected from its most devastating effects than less privileged others. Nobody can observe from the sidelines without being impacted in some way. Nobody gets to sit this one out. Even philosophers who have been, until recently, especially adept at theorizing at an arm's length, have been moving away from ideal theory, and toward engagement with the phenomenologies of lived experience, and with the people caught in the maelstrom. This collection's goal thus became to open up the space for philosophers to speak with all those whose very lives have been upended by the pandemic, and to do so in ways that are intended less to instruct, inform, or problematize, and more to share, to communicate, to connect. In other words, the scholars here are talking to us—to *all* of us. Because, in the end, none of us remain unscathed.

THE PANDEMIC AS (THE STORY OF) TRAUMA

One of the reasons that the pandemic is such a devastating phenomenon is its ongoing traumatic impact on individuals, groups, and entire populations. While all the ways in which its traumas are continuing to dominate our personal and collective consciousness are yet to be explored, what can be said with some certainty is that for the several generations currently in its grip, the world of the "before" and the world of the "after" may never quite line up, and might never constitute the kind of coherent life stories for which we might have hoped.

In a way, trauma is nothing new. From the private catastrophes of accidents, illnesses, abuse, and other losses, to the shared tragedies of war, genocide, socioeconomic upheavals, and political tyranny, we have a sense of what trauma is—of what it does to people—even if for many, much of that knowledge is second-hand, intuited more than directly experienced. But this pandemic—*our* pandemic—is different. Having broken our sense of safety (among those who had such a sense at all) and subverted an inner sense of life's predictability, it also destroyed our means of self-understanding, and our understanding of the world, replacing them with unknown narratives and no-longer-distant horrors. And because, as I have argued elsewhere, this kind of trauma is a totalizing force that unmakes our world, we are left with a kind of world-loss (Gotlib 2020). By world-loss, I do not just mean a loss of freedom to move around, maskless and unworried; I do not just mean the loss of friends and family and relationships; I do not just mean the loss of jobs, of livelihoods, of economic security. Yes, all of these losses matter. But what I think matters in a way that underwrites them all is an all-encompassing loss of the ability to envision and plan one's life, accompanied by a loss of hope that this might *ever* be possible—a loss, in other words, that is not only backward-looking, but forward-looking; a loss of a lifeworld to be experienced, and of lifeworld-constituting stories that grant it meaning. Our reality, our sense of who we are, what our relations to others might be, and, importantly, narratives of what we might yet become, are thus shattered. Instead, trauma leaves us with broken stories that abruptly stop, lacking any further direction, motivation, or in some cases, sense. And, because we are still in the midst of the pandemic, we cannot see a way to reliably reason beyond this narrative break in a way that demarcates an "after." A part of our ongoing trauma, then, has to do with our inability to cope, or to cope well, with the possibility of its endlessness. Are we then defeated by this ongoing trauma? What does being defeated by it actually mean? In other words, even as most of humanity has survived COVID-19, have we at the same time failed in knowing how, and whether, to go on?

In *The Unnamable*, Samuel Beckett tells us that, despite everything, despite every failure and tragedy, we must persist: "You must go on. I can't go on. I'll go on." (Beckett 1965; Brison, 2002b cited in Gotlib 2021). But how? As Susan Brison notes in *Aftermath*, "trauma [. . .] introduces a 'surd'—a nonsensical entry—into the series of events in one's life, making it seem impossible to carry on . . . " (Brison 2002a, 103). What, then, is left when faced with something absurd, with an irrational *something*, after which anything could follow? What stories about who we are and what all of this might mean do we tell now?

Hilde Lindemann has argued that when existing stories about us fail, or fail us, we must tell new ones—better ones (Lindemann 2001). If the surd of the pandemic has rendered our lifeworlds, and the stories through which we create and understand them, no longer accessible or indeed possible, what are these new stories, and how might it be possible to begin telling them?

Perhaps we can begin by considering what does not work. We cannot wish ourselves out of trauma through magical thinking. We cannot simply smile and sloganeer our way out of a pandemic and its many devastations. Applauding essential workers will not make their jobs any safer, or better compensated; displaying "getting back to normal" signs in schools and offices will not bring us any closer to pre-pandemic "normalcy"; removing one's mask while wishing away an airborne virus will not make the virus less virulent or less airborne. What also does not work are static stories that rely on ready-made emplotments—stories that assume that everything will, eventually, be all right, where "all right" means "just as it was before." As I noted elsewhere (Gotlib 2022), "the social critic Barbara Ehrenreich argues in her book *Bright-Sided* (2009), the 'reckless optimism' sold as 'positive thinking' in the United States and elsewhere is just a lie, packaged in gaudy wrapping":

> [W]e cannot levitate ourselves into that blessed condition by wishing it. We need to brace ourselves for a struggle against terrifying obstacles, both of our own making and imposed by the natural world (Ehrenreich 2009).

Instead, we need to unmoor ourselves from some of our past conceptions, perspectives, and plans in order "to be able to rewrite the past in different ways, leading up to an infinite variety of unforeseeable futures" (Brison 2002a, 103). But how do we find these new perspectives—and why does it sometimes seem especially difficult for those who occupy the kinds of privileged social, political, and economic positions that grant the time and space to wonder about this traumatizing predicament to accept the reality of being in the pandemic's grip?

THE PANDEMIC AS DISORIENTING (NEW) PERSPECTIVE

Perhaps it is strange to think of the pandemic as a chance to seek newer perspectives on ourselves, and on our relationships with others and with the world. After all, isolation, fear, and trauma born of historic events might, conceivably, offer no novel stories—maybe no stories at all. Indeed, while social distancing and other forms of isolation have disrupted many of our familiar patterns of socialization and community, these familiar touchstones of our shared humanity have been replaced with anxiety, loneliness, and grief. I suggest that where we find ourselves now is a kind of displacement—or, as philosopher Ami Harbin describes, a kind of moral and practical disorientation (Harbin 2016). We are lost in our traumas, and are experiencing profound existential stuckness, an inability to know how to go on. Indeed,

> [t]hough calls for "social distancing" and "shelter in place" are certainly for our own and the greater good, it is experienced by many of us as a swift and striking change to our daily lived experience—a change that is not of our choosing. The concomitant loss of self is destabilizing and thus traumatic. Moreover, the change is without a clear end in sight, leaving us to wonder what the rest of life might look like. Will this crisis ever end? Anxiety, depression and despair can quickly take hold (Braucher 2020).

But this is not the end of the story: While the pandemic has left virtually no person untouched, its impact has certainly differed among not just individuals, but entire communities. Granted, anxiety, isolation, and fear of a dangerous virus, not to mention the trauma of illness and death itself, do not discriminate, but important differences exist among those for whom COVID-19 trauma meant working from home, childcare challenges, and lack of physical contact with loved ones, and those for whom COVID-19 meant often poorly-protected, dangerous, in-person service work—*essential* work—that made the former's lockdown experiences possible. Thus, the disorientation of the food delivery worker differs, I suggest, from the disorientation of the college professor—and not only because the latter has the privilege of working from home, while the former makes that choice possible. Their disorientations, their traumas, differ in part because of the injustices inherent in our political and socioeconomic systems—where by "our" I mean those from the Global North, broadly construed—structure the background conditions and division of labor in ways that leave large portions of the population much more precarious, much less autonomous, and, at the same time, as the pandemic has revealed for all to see, much more "essential."

Where does this leave us—all of us? On the one hand, we are traumatized as *individual persons*—many of us much more so than others. On the other, we are suddenly forced to see ourselves, and our *necessary connections* through relationships with, and dependencies on, others in startling new ways. What might these reorientations look like? Perhaps those burdened essential workers begin to see more clearly that "essential" ought not be a convenient label created by more privileged others in times of crisis, and demand the kinds of working conditions, compensation, and other terms that reflect the value, the fundamental worth, of their actual labor (in fact, many already are beginning to do just that (Selyukh and Bond 2020)). Perhaps those fortunate enough to experience the pandemic from the relative safety of their homes might begin to view their experiences as opportunities to reconsider, and to shift, what they value, how they value it, and why.

As one belonging to this more privileged category, I have been thinking for some time about how, perhaps especially more recently, human lives have tended not to follow clear, stable, non-disorienting paths. And if some more privileged lives appeared to have been on steadier and more reliable courses, it now seems clear that for many, this was most likely an illusion, or at best a short-term phenomenon. Even if it seems that nothing about this observation is really new—that deep schisms exist, and have always existed, between existentially secure lives and those that are less so—this pandemic nevertheless not only cleared away any lingering debates about these differences, but also reminded those more fortunate that in a global catastrophe, nobody is truly safe from its traumas. Thus, what is needed at this point, I think, is the space to consider, and to reconsider, where we—*all of us*—were, where we have been, and where we might be going. All of the contributors to this volume have done just that: In their own ways, from the perspective of their lived experiences, they have shared this very human, very difficult moment with the readers. I now turn to their contributions.

THE STRUCTURE OF THIS VOLUME

The volume begins with a section entitled "Pandemic Selves," delving into how the pandemic has affected and changed our sense of personal and collective identity. In "The New Normals: Solidarity, Recognition, and Vulnerable Selves in the COVID-19 Pandemic," Vanessa Wills, through both personal narrative and philosophical analysis, explores how COVID-19 has highlighted, transformed, and called into question some of the ways in which we inhabit and experience our bodies, focusing on the ways in which we relate to the vulnerabilities of others. Wills also asks how tensions between individual and social vulnerabilities and agency have shaped, and continue to shape, our experiences of pandemic life. Corey McCall, in "COVID-19 and the Politics of Home," continues the theme of a loss of self and safety by addressing the relationship between home, identity, and the pandemic. He begins with the claim that while "the home is the wellspring of personhood," the current sense of home—now also the locus of our office, childcare work, and other necessary and unexpected functions—has been radically changed as a result of the pandemic, no longer serving as a refuge from the world. McCall then goes on to examine the various dimensions of how the meaning of "home" has changed during the pandemic for differently-situated individuals and groups. J.S. Biehl, in "Waiting to Say Goodbye," closes the section by examining the physical and psychological separation between those dying from the virus and their loved ones. He offers a reflection on this trauma by taking special notice of how it deepens our sense of isolation from those affected. He then considers more generally the value we place on the rituals of parting from those we love for the last time.

The second section, entitled "Pandemic, Illness, and Disability," focuses on facing the complexities, challenges, and, at times, the destructive forces emerging out of the interactions among the pandemic, illness, and disability. In "Sometimes Life Gives You Way Too Many Lemons: An Observation in Nine Parts," Ruth Groenhout offers an uncompromising glimpse into her perspective on the pandemic as a cancer patient. She argues that in addition to her physical illness, "the political cancer" of the (now former) Trump presidency, and the racism, bigotry, hatred and deep injustices into which the nation was collapsing, presents a double burden, and wonders if it is more than one could possibly bear. She asks whether "healing"—in its fullest sense—is possible, and how maybe, just maybe, there might still be some hope among the ruins. In "The Nightmare of Triage and Discrimination: Whose Benefit Is to be Maximized?," Eva Feder Kittay shares her experiences and frustrations in caring for a disabled family member in the middle of a pandemic. She asks why the benefits of disabled people seem to count for so little, and why positive steps to protect them, including those with mental disabilities, is not considered as a part of the overall calculus of just care. She then reminds us that how good a life is—disabled or not—largely depends on a number of factors, not the least of which is the public perception of the value of that life. Concluding this section, Kevin Timpe, in "Disability and Disproportionate Disadvantage," argues that COVID-19 has brought many inequalities that disabled individuals and their families have endured to the forefront. He explores one of those inequalities, namely public education for disabled students during the pandemic (sometimes referred to as "special education"), and suggests that the pandemic clarified how, and to what extent, social challenges disproportionately impact members of already marginalized groups.

Part three, entitled "Pandemic, Precariousness, and Social Justice," centers questions of social justice within the context of the pandemic. In "We Survived COVID-19! (Possibly)," Jamie Lindemann Nelson wonders how—and about what—should philosophers write now? She worries that the existential threat confronting us in Covid-19's wake "is graver than even the loss of many lives; in danger are the structures providing us all with the necessary conditions for living lives about which it makes sense to care, to strive to save and to preserve, to mourn for and to hold in memory." Perhaps, she suggests, in response to the pandemic's suffering and injustices, we might consider not only the role of art, but also pay attention to our responses of grief or mourning. Continuing the theme of surviving pandemic-era injustices, Jennifer Scuro, in "New Labors, New Burdens, Care Work Re-narrated," asks whether, in the middle of the pandemic, helplessness can be understood as both the experience of suffering, as well as a consequence of white saviorism, and whether the labor of thinking about and planning for one's future while disabled is possible in a society that considers disability to be a fate worse than death. Finally, Alexios Alexander, in "Boundaries of Democratic Life in a Time of Pandemic," wonders whether the pandemic created new and powerful sociopolitical and philosophical fault lines, or whether they were already with us. He then examines how a better understanding of freedom and human flourishing, even in the midst of a pandemic, might allow for the reconfiguration of these social and political boundaries.

In the final section of the volume, entitled "Pandemic, Philosophy, and Meaning," the contributors ask how, and whether, philosophy might be able to help us to think through the pandemic and its consequences, and perhaps even to help us to reorient ourselves within our precarious "new normal." In "More Than Mere Survival: Ethical Responsibility and the Intersubjectivity of the Humanities," Claire Elise Katz argues that philosophy is relevant, perhaps even central, to self-understanding—and especially so now, in the midst of a pandemic. She focuses on what philosophy reveals about the tensions between individual rights and our individual and collective responsibilities, as well as on how philosophy as a subset of the humanities clarifies the reasons for which we care about living a flourishing life. Focusing on the challenges of defining a meaningful personal identity while facing post-pandemic anxieties, Barrett Emerick, in "Who Will I Be After All This Is Over?," wonders where things will stand in his life (professionally and otherwise) once the pandemic is over. He addresses the politics of higher education, specifically as it has played out at his own institution, while asking the larger questions about pandemic and post-pandemic uncertainty, belonging, and precarity more broadly. Eyja M. Brynjarsdóttir invites the reader to join her on a kind of a journey in "The COVID-19 Guidebook for Living in an Alternate Universe." She begins with the claim that the pandemic has caused many of us to feel as if the whole world has shifted, bringing with it a feeling of surreality, as if we all became participants in an alternate universe. She then asks the reader to consider the effects of this perhaps unwilling participation on the development and perception of the self. Who are we now, she asks, and which roles are we playing? The section, and the book, conclude with Daniel Conway's "Viral Hope: When Quarantine Comes Home," where he shares his experience teaching *The Plague* by Albert Camus in the midst of the pandemic. Conway examines some of the novel's themes, noting how the meaning of the fictionalized plague intersects with the students' experiences of living through an actual one, focusing specifically on the question of hope. Conway concludes with a discussion of his students' responses and considers whether their real-life predicaments altered their reception of, and experience with, the novel.

CONCLUSION: THIS IS NOT HOW THIS WAS SUPPOSED TO GO

I think that it would not be an overstatement to suggest that all of us, including all of the contributors to this volume, have been at least somewhat surprised, perhaps even shocked, that it is *we* who are living through a world-historical, global pandemic. I have argued elsewhere that perhaps this shock, this "why-us" incredulity that we are in fact the generations to face something so apocalyptic makes up a large part of our traumatized, cognitive-dissonance-like state—where by "our," I mean the privileged, wealthy Global North that has largely been protected both by biomedical interventions and by more socioeconomically secure circumstances from the diseases and epidemics that have plagued the Global South (Gotlib 2021). Another factor in our sense of disbelief is our geographically-limited and historically-impoverished imaginary: we have not seen it happen *here* (at least in most of our lifetimes), and we are much too ignorant of our history to know the prevalence of pandemics even in the not-too-distant past (Gotlib 2021).

But there is another source of our pandemic trauma that has more to do with a failure of our collective imagination. The narrative break of the pandemic created a kind of cognitive dissonance, where our own stories about what a disaster like this pandemic *ought to look like* ran into the brute facts of what our actual pandemic, in fact, *is*. In so many books, on television, in films, and in other corners of popular culture, the stories of our eventual demise predominate: from the Generation X dread of global thermonuclear war of *War Games* and *The Day After*; to the deadly pandemic of *Contagion;* to the apocalypses of *The Day After Tomorrow, The Walking Dead, The Road, 28 Days Later,* and so on, we have learned well the popular narratives of how the end of the world might come, what it would look like—and, importantly, the roles that we, as protagonists (because we are all always protagonists) will play (Gotlib 2021).

And we have imagined the worst: zombie apocalypses, Earth-destroying comets, planetary environmental disaster, and even deadly viruses. In our stories, we—at least some of us—managed to survive, to triumph, to somehow rise above the chaos and destruction. Given all of this psychological, emotional, and imaginative LARPing of the world's end, why are we so traumatized, so shocked, so undone, by our very own pandemic? Why are we not better prepared for the worst-case scenario? Perhaps because

> Covid-19 changed everything. Suddenly, the immense and frightening upheaval, the cataclysm that means nothing can go back to normal, is here, and it's so different from what we imagined. I was expecting *Half-Life*. I was expecting *World War Z*. I've been dressing like I'm in *The Matrix* since 2003. I was not expecting to be facing this sort of thing in snuggly socks and a dressing gown, thousands of miles from home, trying not to panic and craving a proper cup of tea. (Penny 2020)

Where does that leave us? Are we victims, heroes, survivors—or something else? It seems, at least for now, that we are indeed "something else"—unglamorous, traumatized, isolated, anxious survivors. Or else we are the essential workers, battling, aside from the pandemic itself, not ravenous zombies, but our fellow citizens who refuse to do the absolute minimum in the middle of a dangerous virus. Our pandemic is not exciting, it is not a battle between good and evil, it is not a first-person shooter, and it is not a *bildungsroman*: it is an uncertain, fraught attempt at survival—physical, psychological, emotional, social, and professional. It is anything but *The Matrix*. Anything but coherent. Anything but a heroic narrative of eventual triumph. And so we try to make sense of it all—more often than not, we fail at that, too. But we go on. It is with the hope of exploring, engaging with, and perhaps even beginning to understand this shared historical moment, *our* moment, that this volume is offered.

BIBLIOGRAPHY

Beckett, Samuel. *The Unnamable*. New York: Grove Press, 1965.

Braucher, David. "How to Survive 'Social Distancing' and 'Shelter in Place.'" *Psychology Today*, March 22, 2020. Accessed November 5, 2021. https://www.psychologytoday.com/us/blog/life-smarts/202003/how-survive-social-distancing-and-shelter-in-place

Brison, Susan. *Aftermath: Violence and the Remaking of a Self*. Oxford: Princeton University Press. 2002a.

Brison, Susan. "Violence and the Remaking of a Self." The Chronicle of Higher Education, January 18, 2002b. Accessed November 5, 2021. https://www.chronicle.com/article/violence-and-the-remaking-of-a-self/

Ehrenreich, Barbara. *Bright-sided: How the Relentless Promotion of Positive Thinking Has Undermined America*. New York: Metropolitan Books, 2009.

Gotlib, Anna. "Trauma unmakes the world of the self. Can stories repair it?" *Aeon/Psyche,* November 23, 2020. https://psyche.co/ideas/trauma-unmakes-the-world-of-the-self-can-stories-repair-it

Gotlib, Anna. "Letting Go of Familiar Narratives as Tragic Optimism in the Era of COVID-19." *The Journal of Medical Humanities* 42, no. 1 (2021): 81–101. doi:10.1007/s10912-021-09680–8

Gotlib, Anna. "I Remember Damage: Inescapable Scars, Scarring Escapes, and Living with the Absurd." philosophie.ch, March 8, 2022. https://www.philosophie.ch/en/philosophy/articles/2022/2022-03-08-gotlib

Harbin, Ami. *Disorientation and Moral Life*. New York: Oxford University Press, 2016.

Lindemann, Hilde. *Damaged Identities, Narrative Repair*. New York: Cornell University Press, 2001.

Penny, Laurie. "This Is Not the Apocalypse You Were Looking For." *Wired*, March 30, 2020. Accessed on November 5, 2021: https://www.wired.com/story/coronavirus-apocalypse-myths/

Selyukh, Alina, and Shannon Bond. "More Essential Than Ever, Low-Wage Workers Demand More, "April 28, 2020, All Things Considered, *NPR* Accessed on November 5, 2021: https://www.npr.org/2020/04/27/843849435/hometown-heroes-or-whatever-low-wage-workers-want-more-than-praise

PART I

Pandemic Selves

Chapter 1

The New Normals: Solidarity, Recognition, and Vulnerable Selves in the COVID-19 Pandemic

Vanessa Wills

INTRODUCTION

I was living in Munich when, on January 30, 2020, Dr. Tedros Adhanom Gebreyesus, director general of the World Health Organization (WHO), issued a declaration that what was then known as the "novel coronavirus" had come to constitute a "public health emergency of international concern."[1] With this, what later became more widely known as SARS-CoV-2, the virus that causes COVID-19, joined the ranks of such earlier outbreaks as the 2009 spread of H1N1 across international borders and the Zika virus epidemic of 2015 and 2016. For the lay public, this official designation offered some indication of the potential for serious and widespread impacts from COVID-19. However, few then could have foreseen just how pervasive, disruptive, and long-lasting the fallout from this public health emergency of international concern would become.

On January 28, 2020, two days before the WHO's declaration, local Munich news reports carried word that Bavarian health officials had confirmed the first known case in Germany of a patient stricken with disease by the novel coronavirus.[2] This strange illness that had made its way close to us began to come up as a topic of conversation among my friends there, but it still felt quite abstract.

Three days after the WHO's declaration, on February 2, 2020, I boarded a plane to Washington, DC. There, I was with my students at the George Washington University face-to-face for just a few scant weeks before the public health emergency of international concern blossomed into a large-scale, imminent, and mortal global threat, overwhelming hospitals worldwide, emptying the streets in metropoles, and shuttering university buildings on the campus where I teach.

Commentators have drawn parallels to the AIDS crisis of the 1980s and to the polio epidemic of the 1950s.[3] These are some of the most apt and striking parallels to be found in any of our living historical memories. But with the exception of a few centenarians born onto a globe ravaged by world war and the 1918 flu pandemic, no one living on the planet today has ever been witness to the global spread of fatal and disabling communicable illness on anything like the current scale—one to which we have rapidly become strangely accustomed. If we have little in the way of parallel or precedent to help us make sense of this experience, then it must also be noted that we have still less in the way of critical distance from which we might stand to reflect upon the pandemic's effect on our perceptions, our habits, and our relationships to ourselves, to one another, and to the world. It is typically hindsight that brings wisdom, which is why it has been said that the Owl of Minerva spreads its wings at dusk. As I write, it is clearly not even noontime.

What is already clear as the day just begins to break on this disaster, and what was clear even in those first uncertain weeks and months of 2020, is that COVID-19 is not simply a biological illness that can beset and destroy particular bodies, but a complex of systemic social failures that have colluded to produce something very much like the worst-case scenario. Without widespread poverty; without lack of healthcare; without racist, ableist, and classist notions rendering some lives wholly expendable; without capitalism's insistence that short-term profits trump human well-being; without imperialism and antagonism among nation-states; without systematic miseducation and abuse of reason; and without the facile opposition of individual liberty to social responsibility, it is difficult to imagine that the novel coronavirus would have snowballed into the global threat it has become.

It is true in principle, of course, that every human person has a body and that therefore every human person is vulnerable to biological assault just by virtue of having a body that is delicately and intricately arranged in the way that bodies are. Every human being can become infected with SARS-CoV-2 and become sickened with COVID-19. In reality, however, each human body is socially, economically, politically, and geographically located in ways that significantly determine that body's susceptibility to neglect and harm in general and to the ravages of the pandemic in particular.

In this way, the pandemic highlights the significance of feminist theory's concept of "embodiment" as well as classical Marxist theory's categories of "alienation" (failure to recognize ourselves as ourselves) and "exploitation" (the extraction of value). We—humanity—are engaged in a peculiar failure to recognize ourselves in differently embodied others. Still less do we fully consider what the pandemic makes fully clear: Our fate depends on one another. Attending to the frailties and vulnerabilities of each of our own particular bodies requires that we be motivated by an affect of care toward the bodies of others. My own body, being Black, female, and chronically ill, is one whose ostensibly "low" worth is clearly marked out as overdetermined in mainstream pandemic rhetoric, even as economic and educational privilege allow me greater resources to protect it than others have to protect theirs. Rather than emphasize care for others, much pandemic discourse has encouraged the attitude that COVID-19 is an illness only affecting "those bodies over there."

On February 1, 2020, two days after the WHO declared COVID-19 to be a "public health emergency of international concern," I visited the Dachau Concentration Camp Memorial Site, located just south of Munich. Almost every weekend, for months, I had contemplated going, and every weekend until my very last one in Germany, I thought to myself, "Perhaps next weekend." But I did find myself a visitor there, as I knew I would and as I had previously visited the memorial sites at Sachsenhausen and Buchenwald. At Dachau, I found myself struck by the brutal and insistent reduction of human beings to their exploitability, to what—their homes, their labor, their teeth—could be extracted from them and accumulated.

My intention in the following pages is to explore how COVID-19 has highlighted, transformed, and called into question some of the ways in which we inhabit our bodies, experience our bodies, and are our bodies, as well as some of the ways in which we relate to the vulnerable bodies of others. I do this through a mixture of personal narrative, critical reflections on the broader social context, and engagement with media reports and scholarly literature. I address a set of four paired themes. These are: Embodiment and Disability, Social Distance and the "Bubble," Self-Care and Essential Labor, and Masking and the New Normals. My aim in addressing these themes is to articulate how a tension and a dialectic of individual and social vulnerability, as well as of individual and social rationality and of individual and social agency, has so far shaped our experience of pandemic life.

EMBODIMENT AND DISABILITY

They're not sick unless they're dying . . . Who are these people?

—Trout Fishing in America, "Who Are These People?"[4]

It was a strange thing to leave Germany, whose social safety net is somewhat tattered by decades of neoliberal assault but remains more or less intact with respect to public health, and to prepare to weather the pandemic in the laissez-faire health environment of the United States. In place of any coherent strategy to deliver care, there was an oft-repeated message meant to reassure: COVID-19 is only likely to kill or seriously sicken the elderly and those with "preexisting conditions," the unspoken addendum being that these people were about as good as dead already, so whether it was COVID-19 or something else that ushered them those last few steps through death's door was of little real consequence in the grand scheme of things.

As a person with a "preexisting condition," I quickly realized that I was one of those people considered to be already about as good as dead. Only I was very much alive, and I wished to remain so. The same is true for all the elderly, chronically ill, disabled, and/or immunocompromised and immunosuppressed people that I knew. For me and for others with similarly situated bodies, the "reassurance"—both the advice itself and the gladness and relief with which it was widely met—felt like terrifying confirmation that we were on our own to survive the pandemic. A response to COVID-19 that took our deaths as a given would be considered socially palatable.[5]

The irony of this is twofold. First, in the United States, the messaging around COVID-19 as a disease that only affected the already vulnerable fostered a complacency that in turn helped to fuel a lackadaisical approach to suppressing the spread of the disease. People die from the flu every year, we heard, and we don't stop everything and take emergency measures to prevent that from happening. We calculate it as an "acceptable" loss and get on. If COVID-19 was just a "bad flu" that was only likely to kill those who were less economically productive in any case, then perhaps, as the dominant thinking seemed to be in those first weeks, we should approach it just as we do the flu and its victims. So even with the dire warnings from China, and even as Italy was besieged by plague, in the United States, public policy virtually guaranteed the spread of the disease. There were no calls for social distancing to mitigate the spread of this "bad flu" until March, and the Centers for Disease Control did not recommend face masks until April 2020, more than two months after the WHO's January 30 warning.

Second, the social failure to regard "the disabled" as an unstable category, one whose extension could expand, helped to fuel a strange hyperfocus just on who was or was not likely to be killed by COVID-19. There was—and at the time of this writing, still is—very little serious public discussion of the SARS-CoV-2 virus's capacity to render disabled and chronically ill those previously considered "healthy" and able-bodied.[6]

It is already surreal to observe as your society takes your chronically ill and disabled condition to be some sad misfortune rendering your death barely worth expending any effort to prevent. It is still more surreal to observe this while so many apparently able-bodied people appear curiously indifferent as to whether they themselves might become disabled by COVID-19 and wind up in the exact same condition they find so pitiable in you. The social erasure of disability leaves the pages of mainstream discourse so threadbare, right where there should be some conversation about how we care for the unwell, that becoming disabled hardly appears as a possibility even though almost all of us will experience this at some point in our lives. As the phenomenon of "long COVID" has shown us, one might start out without any "preexisting condition" at all and then later acquire one that remains, stubborn, intractable. But as the silence around long COVID has also shown, those who contracted COVID-19 and did not die, but also did not become well, seem to have joined the ranks of the forgotten and expendable.

As a chronically ill person living through the COVID-19 pandemic, I have found myself in a curious position. I must both insist that my life is worth preserving, which it is, while at the same time I look on with horror and confusion at the braggadocio with which so many seem to court an infection that might make their lives more like mine. Surely, I think, they'd avoid that if they knew. But the indifference is not only an individual attitude; it is a social bargain. The logic of COVID policy in the United States is the logic of flu outbreaks is the logic of driving human beings to their graves through overwork. We don't stop everything and take emergency measures when people die from lack of healthcare or when families don't have water or when children die of malnutrition, as they do every day. There was, I quickly came to see, a certain naivete in expecting the response to COVID-19 to look any different at all without a fight. The horror of commanding human beings to "sacrifice themselves for the economy" was nothing other than the horror of quotidian capitalism taken to its logical conclusion in a time of crisis.[7]

SOCIAL DISTANCE AND THE "BUBBLE"

A key element of the pandemic's eerie horror has been the sudden imposition of stifling physical isolation as the most effective means by which to stop its spread. The need for "social distance" has created a kind of double whammy of trauma, on the one hand, and lack of access to the social networks and forms of togetherness we most rely upon to process that trauma, on the other.

In the most extreme expression of this, the COVID-19 pandemic instills not only a fear of death but specifically the terror of dying a "bad" death; that is to say, a fear of dying miserable, afraid, and alone. A March 16, 2020, article in the *New York Times* reported that in Italy, "[f]amily members are spirited away and, because of the danger of contagion, often die in the hospital isolation without any family or friends around."[8] In November 2020, an article in the *Journal of Bioethical Inquiry* noted, "When patients need their loved ones most—when they are scared, critically ill, or dying—loved ones are not allowed to be with them."[9]

Those who could do so were implored to self-isolate and to establish their "bubble," a small cell of trusted people with whom to ride out the pandemic together for however indefinitely long that might be necessary. City ordinances were written to establish which kinds of social interaction were permissible and which were banned as dangerous frivolities, often limiting permissible social interactions to cohabitants or to members of officially recognized "families" of legally married couples or of parents, children, and siblings organized into nuclear family arrangements.[10] It was frequently ambiguous whether friends and lovers who relied on one another for social support, but whose connection lacked official sanction, were breaking the law every time they visited one another in their homes.

Like many other chronically ill people, I found my friends' anxiety and upset about home isolation curious and difficult to comprehend at first. I had long since become accustomed to my body's vicissitudes, which might suddenly, out of nowhere, confine me to my room through pain and disability. I knew exactly what to do as it became clear that home isolation would be necessary; just as I know how to respond to my body's signs, in my bones and on my skin, that I must prepare to withdraw. I knew what to buy, how to organize my home, and how to pass the days. What's more, I was able to give advice to those for whom extended home isolation with no obvious end in sight was a thoroughly unique experience. Such disruptions had long before become so familiar to my routine that it was jarring to be reminded that sudden forced physical isolation was not "normal."

One saving grace of a twenty-first-century pandemic has been the availability of technological media through which to reestablish, maintain, and deepen connections. Like many others, I found myself reconnecting with friends I hadn't spoken to in years and establishing more routine communication with those I had been in touch with only sparsely and intermittently. At the same time, some connections began to wither under the strain of real or perceived physical distance and the mental health challenges of fear, crisis, and isolation.

Yet my capacity to isolate and keep myself safe was thoroughly premised on others' exposure to harm because we live in a society that makes public health into a zero-sum game. I had groceries delivered. I ordered supplies online. I used food delivery apps. There seemed to be no obvious "right" answer about how to navigate a thousand ethical quandaries. I think now that it seemed that way because there really was no one "right" answer, whether obvious or otherwise. Go to the store yourself and you are one more body possibly carrying contagion to others. Stay home, and you are exercising your privilege to stay safe while benefiting from others' lack of privilege to do the same. If we had a rational system, then local governments would step in, with the guidance of public health authorities, to help organize the delivery of food and necessities to people at home in ways that are both safe and equitable. As it was, people without the individual private means to self-isolate frequently found themselves in crowded, and often unsanitary, work conditions without personal protective equipment, their health sacrificed for profit.

SELF-CARE AND ESSENTIAL LABOR

> [*Max Stirner*] *believes that the communists want to "make sacrifices" for "society," when they want at most to sacrifice existing society . . . their struggle is the common cause of all people who have outgrown the bourgeois system as a sacrifice that they make to themselves.*
>
> —Karl Marx, *Critique of the German Ideology*[11]

As for so many others, one of my initial responses to the pandemic was to take the opportunity for outdoor recreation, as "essential exercise" remained a permissible reason to leave one's home even under the emergency city ordinances. There was so much that no one could do anymore, or at least not safely. Even being outside at all felt like an incredible risk, as in the early months of 2020, we still knew little about how SARS-CoV-2 spread. Was it something you caught through contact with infected surfaces, and if so, how long did surfaces remain infectious? Could it linger in the fresh air long after an infected person had left one city block and moved on to another? City life, usually a source of excitement, contact, and connection, suddenly transformed from bustling streets to nervous individuals walking in ones and sometimes twos, fearfully keeping six feet apart from any passing stranger. And yet, to be outside, to move my body, to breathe in fresh air—even if through a mask, even if with the then-incalculable risk of contracting the virus—seemed a necessary counterbalance to the monotony of the indoors as weeks dragged on. Lockdown's sudden impact on physical activity levels no doubt contributed to the mental strain of pandemic life. A July 2021 study of healthcare workers in Singapore, for example, found that "healthcare workers with the highest rates of depressive symptoms were those who had reported a three-day reduction in their weekly physical activity frequency" during lockdown.[12]

In lockdown, the challenge of caring for my body became something of a minefield. Regular exercise helps me to maintain my strength, flexibility, and mobility and to stave off pain and disability, but getting outside to exercise felt risky in all the ways just enumerated. I developed a terror of going to the doctor, where I would be indoors and not socially distanced from health professionals; in any case, most doctors were not seeing patients in person. As is the case for many people with chronic illness, my flare-ups are often triggered by stress; as I thought constantly about how to keep myself and my loved ones safe as the world seemed to burn, my stress was through the roof and became one more crisis to manage.

In the end, with so many unknowns, I embraced as my touchstone the thing I knew about how to keep myself well and pushed past my trepidation to get outside and walk. But not long after I established a regular walking routine, I developed joint pain so severe that I soon found myself constricted by it, less and less able to walk any distance from my home. I was no stranger to severe and chronic pain, but this felt very different from my normal baseline of bodily discomfort. Eventually, by early fall 2020, the pain and disability had become so severe that I could not sleep through the night. I had to overcome my hesitation and be seen by a doctor, who diagnosed me with end-stage osteoarthritis in my left hip. I would have to have it replaced.

"Self-care," the thing I was struggling to figure out while inside a body that seemed to thwart my best attempts, has been a watchword of pandemic life. Of course, self-care had never before seemed quite so necessary as it did in lockdown. There was no public, social care and the private caregiving of family and friends that typically fills that void was suddenly unavailable for many due to the requirements of social distancing. Self-care was often the only kind of care one had available, and even that existed in a highly constrained, commoditized form.[13] Peloton, a maker of high-end exercise bikes, saw record sales.[14] It seems that everyone with access to the kitchen equipment to do so became a baker.[15] Home decor sales in the United States soared.

Even amid the widespread isolation and atomization of life in lockdown, the "essential workers" whose labor had only become more hazardous, more backbreaking, and more exploitative broke out from the logic of self-care as another commodity to be sold. The Instacart workers delivering baking goods to affluent homes, the Amazon employees packaging scented candles and sweatpants, the dockworkers facilitating the entry of goods from factories overseas—all organized and, in many cases, struck, for better pay, better benefits, better workplace safety, and better access to PPE.[16] By some counts, 2020 saw the highest number of wildcat strikes in many years. A groundswell of labor activism swept across the United States as workers whose labor had finally been recognized as "essential" in word demanded that it also be recognized as essential in deed—that they and their work be valued and that they have the means to do their jobs safely and to protect themselves and their families.

This labor activism, often led by Black and Brown workers who were some of the hardest hit by the pandemic, laid the groundwork for the largest US civil rights uprising in decades: the Black Lives Matter protests catalyzed by the brutal state killing of George Floyd. Led by the poor and working people who never had the opportunity to isolate or to social distance, whose only bid for safety and self-care could come in the form of mass action, tens of thousands of people in the United States and worldwide poured into the street, marching, rallying, and protesting a system that had made its priorities, and its utter incapacity to satisfy human needs, very clear.

That was in June 2020. I didn't know yet that my left hip was broken, that it had crumbled away to almost nothing. What I did know for certain was that it was painful and unreliable, trapping me at home. And that even if the hip hadn't prevented me from getting out into the street with the protestors, my immunocompromised status would have made it unwise.

I had thankfully long since resolved the feelings of resentment for my body that I felt when I was younger. Why should I be angry at my body for being sick? Together we are simply doing our best. But the combination of lockdown and disability did cause me to feel disconnected from it in a way that I thought I had also overcome. With little to stave off the existential dread, I threw myself into my work: teaching remotely, editing a journal, doing research, and writing both academic and public philosophy. I worked constantly. I knew that it was unsustainable, but it was the most reliable way I knew to avoid falling into despair. I was thankful, and still am, to have work that I knew was valuable. While I was working, I never questioned whether my time was well spent, whether my life mattered to others, whether it was better that I survive the pandemic or be allowed to become one of its casualties.

It is hard to disentangle the meaning I found in work from the productivist ideology of capitalism. But knowing that my work gave me clarity in the midst of chaos and crisis that I was then able to share with others gave my days meaning. Doing work that was grounded in, guided by, and in aid of mass working-class struggle for a world based on human care for one another was, for me, a kind of touchstone. It helped me to resolve a real tension between the false appearances of "self-care" as private consumerist egoism, and "essential labor" as a self-abnegating sacrifice to "the economy," some strange, hungry master commanding humanity to its death.

CONCLUSION: MASKING AND THE NEW NORMALS

Because I have access to high-quality healthcare, my chronic illness and disability are well treated and controlled. They are therefore typically "invisible." As my hip deteriorated in lockdown, I had the strange experience of my disability becoming both more and less visible. I walked with a pronounced limp and eventually used a cane, but since my employment responsibilities had transitioned to a remote format, I was rarely seen attempting to move myself around. I taught my classes and delivered scholarly presentations, but I was able to do all of this sitting down more or less comfortably in my own home. Hardly anyone except those closest to me saw that I was struggling physically. This offered me the opportunity to keep my pain and disability mostly "invisible" if I wanted to: to mask it. As challenging as lockdown was, I was much more able to remain active and engaged with my work than I might have been had I experienced the same health challenge a year earlier.

That same access to healthcare meant that in March 2021, I was able to have the total hip replacement surgery that I desperately needed. After a long recovery, people who see me now are shocked to learn I had the surgery at all; to look at me, you would never know except perhaps by my scar. It was also in March 2021 that I received my second dose of a COVID vaccine. With a new hip and a new immunity to SARS-CoV-2, I waited eagerly for summer and for the world to begin to "reopen."

The university buildings are open again. There is no social distancing, but everyone on campus is "vaxxed and masked." The restaurants are packed with diners. The city streets have stirred back to life. So much has returned to some semblance of "normal," and yet what the pandemic has exposed about the conflict between capitalism's death drive and human beings' wish to be safe, healthy, and alive remains out in the open in a way it wasn't always before. We see it expressed, for example, in the so-called Great Resignation.[17] With even just a little economic relief, workers are increasingly "voting with their feet" and rejecting low-paid, grueling, demoralizing, and often unsafe work. The pressure to mask basic human needs and frailties, to pretend they aren't there and are irrelevant to workplace demands on employees, is for now no longer tenable in the way it was in a pre-COVID environment. Workers' response to a lessening of the economic pressure to place their lives on the line for capital reveals something of the extent to which the "free market" is founded entirely in coercion.

The irony of continuing widespread skepticism about the vaccine as a kind of "secret government plot" is that the real government plot is right out there in the open. The "plot," which no politician or CEO can be accused of attempting to conceal, is to resist the kind of total social transformation that would be necessary in order to afford human lives the value with which they should be treated. The "plot" is instead to embrace a bare-bones, vaccine-only public health policy, and to push the world as quickly as possible back onto the same track that led us into this crisis in the first place. The "plot" is to deny, as far as possible, the obvious truth that vaccines are only a start, that individual pharmaceutical solutions to a public health crisis are necessary but can only get us so far, as surging COVID-19 cases across Europe and the United States in the late fall of 2021 make clear.[18]

Living through this pandemic while navigating a personal health crisis that intersected with it and did not allow me to simply put my own vulnerability out of mind has been a harrowing but eye-opening experience. In some ways, I was more isolated than ever before. In other ways, it was novel and affirming, and bred solidarity with others who seemed to understand more about how the bizarre "normal" of pandemic life was not entirely abnormal for me. And it placed me in a position to offer these reflections that I hope may be useful to others.

The crisis has not passed, and we cannot yet speak from a place of hindsight on this awful chapter. To pause and reflect upon how the story is developing so far is nonetheless a worthwhile exercise, especially as it has already revealed so much about our collective capacity to shape how the rest of it unfolds.

BIBLIOGRAPHY

Anderson-Shaw, Lisa K., and Fred A. Zar. "COVID-19, Moral Conflict, Distress, and Dying Alone." *Journal of Bioethical Inquiry* 17, no. 4 (2020): 777–82.

Arcieri, Amanda A. "The Relationships between COVID-19 Anxiety, Ageism, and Ableism." *Psychological Reports* (2021): 00332941211018404.

Böhmer, Merle M., Udo Buchholz, Victor M. Corman, Martin Hoch, Katharina Katz, Durdica V. Marosevic, Stefanie Böhm, et al. "Investigation of a COVID-19 Outbreak in Germany Resulting from a Single Travel-Associated Primary Case: A Case Series." *Lancet Infectious Diseases* 20, no. 8 (2020): 920–28.

Cassidy, K. "Ableism's Hand in the Perpetuation of a Pandemic." San Francisco AIDS Foundation, May 19, 2021. https://www.sfaf.org/collections/beta/ableisms-hand-in-the-perpetuation-of-a-pandemic/.

Clifford, Catherine. "Why Everyone Is #QuarantineBaking Their Way through the Coronavirus Pandemic." CNBC, March 28, 2020. https://www.cnbc.com/2020/03/27/coronavirus-why-everyone-is-baking-their-way-through-the-pandemic.html.

Corder, Mike. "Not out of the Woods: COVID Cases Rising in Western Europe." AP News, November 12, 2021. https://apnews.com/article/coronavirus-pandemic-lifestyle-germany-europe-western-europe-be9a84ddaf7b9b3cc927d47428683201.

Ellenberg, Susan S., and Jeffrey S. Morris. "AIDS and COVID: A Tale of Two Pandemics and the Role of Statisticians." *Statistics in Medicine* 40, no. 11 (2021): 2499–510.

Deliso, Meredith. "Vermont Has the Highest Vaccination Rate in the Country. So Why Are Cases Surging?" ABC News, November 12, 2021. https://abcnews.go.com/Health/vermont-highest-vaccination-rate-country-cases-surging/story?id=81090116.

District of Columbia. Mayor's Order 2020–063. April 15, 2020. https://coronavirus.dc.gov/sites/default/files/dc/sites/coronavirus/publication/attachmentsMayorsOrder2020.063.pdf.

Elk, Mike. "How Black & Brown Workers Are Redefining Strikes in the Digital COVID Age." *Payday Report*, July 8, 2020. https://paydayreport.com/how-black-brown-workers-are-redefining-strikes-in-a-digital-covid-age/.

Hammerly, Allison. "Then and Now: Polio and COVID-19." *Perspectives*, fall 2020. https://cvm.msu.edu/news/perspectives-magazine/perspectives-fall-2020/then-and-now-polio-and-covid-19.

Hickson, Michael. "Ableism and Quality of Life during the Coronavirus Pandemic." *Journal of Hospital Medicine* 16, no. 5 (2021).

Horowitz, Jason, and Emma Bubola. "Italy's Coronavirus Victims Face Death Alone, with Funerals Postponed." *New York Times*, March 16, 2020. https://www.nytimes.com/2020/03/16/world/europe/italy-coronavirus-funerals.html.

Idlet, Ezra, and Keith Grimwood (writing together as the band Trout Fishing in America). "Who Are These People?" *Who Are These People*? Trout Records, 1994.

Knodel, Jamie. "Texas Lt. Gov. Dan Patrick Suggests He, Other Seniors Willing to Die to Get Economy Going." NBC News, March 24, 2020. https://www.nbcnews.com/news/us-news/texas-lt-gov-dan-patrick-suggests-he-other-seniors-willing-n1167341.

Kua, Zaylea, Fadzil Hamzah, Pei T. Tan, Li J. Ong, Benedict Tan, and Zhongwei Huang. "Physical Activity Levels and Mental Health Burden of Healthcare Workers during COVID-19 Lockdown." *Stress and Health*, 2021.

Marx, Karl, and Friedrich Engels. *Critique of the German Ideology* in *Marx & Engels Collected Works*, Vol 5: *Marx and Engels: 1845–1847*. New York: Lawrence and Wishart, 1976.

Oladipo, Gloria. "'It's a Sweat Factory': Instacart Workers Ready to Strike for Pay and Conditions." *Guardian*, October 15, 2021. https://www.theguardian.com/business/2021/oct/15/instacart-workers-strike-pay.

Perego, Elisa, Felicity Callard, Laurie Stras, Barbara Melville-Jóhannesson, Rachel Pope, and Nisreen A. Alwan. "Why the Patient-Made Term 'Long COVID Is Needed." *Wellcome Open Research* 5, no. 224 (2020): 224.

Pisani, Joseph. "Amazon Faces Biggest Union Push in its History." AP News, March 29, 2021. https://apnews.com/article/amazon-workers-union-c8493c24dabe7609de8fec8716460737.

Pulrang, Andrew. "What Disabled People Are Thinking and Feeling about the Pandemic, One Year Later." *Forbes*, March 21, 2021. https://www.forbes.com/sites

/andrewpulrang/2021/03/21/what-disabled-people-are-thinking-and-feeling-about-the-pandemic-one-year-later/?sh=2408d1453277.

Puzio, Angelica. "Have We Been Doing Self-Care All Wrong?" *Washington Post*, October 1, 2021. https://www.washingtonpost.com/lifestyle/wellness/self-care-meaning-history/2021/10/01/c4f8a1ea-2232-11ec-9309-b743b79abc59_story.html.

Sharma, Priya, Sumit Bharti, and Isha Garg. "Post COVID Fatigue: Can We Really Ignore It?" *Indian Journal of Tuberculosis*, 2021.

Thomas, Lauren. "Peloton Says Recent Spike in COVID-19 Cases, Lockdowns Are Boosting Sales." CNBC, November 5, 2020. https://www.cnbc.com/2020/11/05/peloton-says-recent-spike-in-covid-19-cases-lockdowns-boosting-sales.html.

Thompson, Derek. "The Great Resignation Is Accelerating." *Atlantic*, October 15, 2021. https://www.theatlantic.com/ideas/archive/2021/10/great-resignation-accelerating/620382/.

Tierney, John. "Unlearned AIDS Lessons for COVID." *Wall Street Journal*, October 3, 2021. https://www.wsj.com/articles/aids-panic-covid-19-coronavirus-pandemic-experts-politicized-fauci-follow-science-11633290650.

World Health Organization. "2019-nCoV Outbreak Is an Emergency of International Concern." January 31, 2020. https://www.euro.who.int/en/health-topics/health-emergencies/pages/news/news/2020/01/2019-ncov-outbreak-is-an-emergency-of-international-concern.

Yong, Ed. "Long-Haulers Are Fighting for Their Future." *Atlantic*, September 1, 2021. https://www.theatlantic.com/science/archive/2021/09/covid-19-long-haulers-pandemic-future/619941/.

NOTES

1. World Health Organization, "2019-nCoV Outbreak Is an Emergency of International Concern," January 31, 2020, https://www.euro.who.int/en/health-topics/health-emergencies/pages/news/news/2020/01/2019-ncov-outbreak-is-an-emergency-of-international-concern.

2. Merle M. Böhmer, Udo Buchholz, Victor M. Corman, Martin Hoch, Katharina Katz, Durdica V. Marosevic, Stefanie Böhm, et al., "Investigation of a COVID-19 Outbreak in Germany Resulting from a Single Travel-Associated Primary Case: A Case Series," *Lancet Infectious Diseases* 20, no. 8 (2020): 920–28.

3. Susan S. Ellenberg and Jeffrey S. Morris, "AIDS and COVID: A Tale of Two Pandemics and the Role of Statisticians," *Statistics in Medicine* 40, no. 11 (2021): 2499–510; John Tierney, "Unlearned AIDS Lessons for COVID," *Wall Street Journal*, October 3, 2021, https://www.wsj.com/articles/aids-panic-covid-19-coronavirus-pandemic-experts-politicized-fauci-follow-science-11633290650; Allison Hammerly, "Then and Now: Polio and COVID-19," *Perspectives*, fall 2020, https://cvm.msu.edu/news/perspectives-magazine/perspectives-fall-2020/then-and-now-polio-and-covid-19.

4. Ezra Idlet and Keith Grimwood (writing together as the band Trout Fishing in America), "Who Are These People?" *Who Are These People*? (Trout Records, 1994).

5. Michael Hickson, "Ableism and Quality of Life during the Coronavirus Pandemic," *Journal of Hospital Medicine* 16, no. 5 (2021); Andrew Pulrang, "What Disabled People Are Thinking and Feeling about the Pandemic, One Year Later," *Forbes*, March 21, 2021, https://www.forbes.com/sites/andrewpulrang/2021/03/21/what-disabled-people-are-thinking-and-feeling-about-the-pandemic-one-year-later/?sh=2408d1453277; Amanda A. Arcieri, "The Relationships between COVID-19 Anxiety, Ageism, and Ableism," *Psychological Reports* (2021): 00332941211018404; K. Cassidy, "Ableism's Hand in the Perpetuation of a Pandemic," San Francisco AIDS Foundation, May 19, 2021, https://www.sfaf.org/collections/beta/ableisms-hand-in-the-perpetuation-of-a-pandemic/.

6. Elisa Perego, Felicity Callard, Laurie Stras, Barbara Melville-Jóhannesson, Rachel Pope, and Nisreen A. Alwan, "Why the Patient-Made Term 'Long COVID Is Needed," *Wellcome Open Research* 5, no. 224 (2020): 224; Priya Sharma, Sumit Bharti, and Isha Garg, "Post COVID Fatigue: Can We Really Ignore It?" *Indian Journal of Tuberculosis*, 2021; Ed Yong, "Long-Haulers Are Fighting for Their Future," *Atlantic*, September 1, 2021, https://www.theatlantic.com/science/archive/2021/09/covid-19-long-haulers-pandemic-future/619941/.

7. Jamie Knodel, "Texas Lt. Gov. Dan Patrick Suggests He, Other Seniors Willing to Die to Get Economy Going," NBC News, March 24, 2020, https://www.nbcnews.com/news/us-news/texas-lt-gov-dan-patrick-suggests-he-other-seniors-willing-n1167341. Infamously, the lieutenant governor of Texas expressed his view, on behalf of every person over the age of seventy, that they ought to be willing to die of COVID rather than have measures be taken to protect seniors that might impact profits.

8. Jason Horowitz and Emma Bubola, "Italy's Coronavirus Victims Face Death Alone, with Funerals Postponed," *New York Times*, March 16, 2020, https://www.nytimes.com/2020/03/16/world/europe/italy-coronavirus-funerals.html.

9. Lisa K. Anderson-Shaw and Fred A. Zar, "COVID-19, Moral Conflict, Distress, and Dying Alone," *Journal of Bioethical Inquiry* 17, no. 4 (2020): 777–82.

10. Washington, DC's April 15, 2020, "Stay At Home" order, for example, required that "if leaving their residence, all individuals must continue to social distance from others not in their household."

11. Karl Marx and Friedrich Engels, *Critique of the German Ideology* in *Marx & Engels Collected Works*, Vol 5: *Marx and Engels: 1845–1847* (New York: Lawrence and Wishart, 1976).

12. Zaylea Kua, Fadzil Hamzah, Pei T. Tan, Li J. Ong, Benedict Tan, and Zhongwei Huang, "Physical Activity Levels and Mental Health Burden of Healthcare Workers during COVID-19 Lockdown," *Stress and Health*, 2021.

13. Angelica Puzio, "Have We Been Doing Self-Care All Wrong?" *Washington Post*, October 1, 2021, https://www.washingtonpost.com/lifestyle/wellness/self-care-meaning-history/2021/10/01/c4f8a1ea-2232-11ec-9309-b743b79abc59_story.html.

14. Lauren Thomas, "Peloton Says Recent Spike in COVID-19 Cases, Lockdowns Are Boosting Sales," CNBC, November 5, 2020, https://www.cnbc.com/2020/11/05/peloton-says-recent-spike-in-covid-19-cases-lockdowns-boosting-sales.html.

15. Catherine Clifford, "Why Everyone Is #QuarantineBaking Their Way through the Coronavirus Pandemic," CNBC, March 28, 2020, https://www.cnbc.com/2020/03/27/coronavirus-why-everyone-is-baking-their-way-through-the-pandemic.html.

16. Mike Elk, "How Black & Brown Workers Are Redefining Strikes in the Digital COVID Age," *Payday Report*, July 8, 2020, https://paydayreport.com/how-black-brown-workers-are-redefining-strikes-in-a-digital-covid-age/; Joseph Pisani, "Amazon Faces Biggest Union Push in its History," AP News, March 29, 2021, https://apnews.com/article/amazon-workers-union-c8493c24dabe7609de8fec8716460737; Gloria Oladipo, "'It's a Sweat Factory': Instacart Workers Ready to Strike for Pay and Conditions," *Guardian*, October 15, 2021, https://www.theguardian.com/business/2021/oct/15/instacart-workers-strike-pay.

17. Derek Thompson, "The Great Resignation Is Accelerating," *Atlantic*, October 15, 2021, https://www.theatlantic.com/ideas/archive/2021/10/great-resignation-accelerating/620382/.

18. Meredith Deliso, "Vermont Has the Highest Vaccination Rate in the Country. So Why Are Cases Surging?" ABC News, November 12, 2021, https://abcnews.go.com/Health/vermont-highest-vaccination-rate-country-cases-surging/story?id=81090116; Mike Corder, "Not out of the Woods: COVID Cases Rising in Western Europe," AP News, November 12, 2021, https://apnews.com/article/coronavirus-pandemic-lifestyle-germany-europe-western-europe-be9a84ddaf7b9b3cc927d47428683201.

Chapter 2

COVID-19 and the Politics of Home

Corey McCall

In early 2020, people throughout the world suddenly found themselves confined to their homes. In the final months of 2019, news outlets began reporting on a dangerous new virus in China, and by January 2020, Chinese authorities had imposed quarantines in Wuhan Province in an attempt to stem the spread of a new deadly disease. Other national governments, first in Europe and subsequently in North America, would soon follow suit as the disease spread throughout their populations. People found themselves virtual prisoners in their homes, and hence began to experience their homes differently than they had before these pandemic-imposed quarantines. Here is how sociologist Matthew Desmond characterized the meaning of home in the epilogue to his book *Evicted*:

> The home is the center of life. It is a refuge from the grind of work, the pressure of school, and the menace of the streets. We say that at home, we can "be ourselves." Everywhere else, we are someone else. At home, we remove our masks.
>
> The home is the wellspring of personhood. It is where our identity takes root and blossoms, where as children, we imagine, play, and question, and as adolescents, we retreat and try. As we grow older, we hope to raise a family or pursue work. When we try to understand ourselves, we often begin by considering the kind of home in which we were raised.[1]

Desmond published his influential study of US housing policies in 2016. The epilogue, "Home and Hope" describes how Americans typically experience "home" that is likely familiar to many of his readers. He begins the epilogue with this somewhat hackneyed conception of home in order to show how this dream has become unrealizable for many of the individuals profiled in his study. Indeed, Desmond focuses on the experience of renters in Milwaukee to show just how precarious this lived experience of home has become for many Americans. My purpose in citing the opening passages of his epilogue differs somewhat from Desmond's, for I believe we can recognize in this litany of the nostalgic meanings people typically associate with "home" just how much our sense of home has changed as a result of the pandemic.

While the home certainly remained the center of life for many Americans during the pandemic, it lost its sense of a refuge from the world. Early in the pandemic, the metaphorical masks that people removed upon arriving home in Desmond's vision became literal as individuals tried to protect themselves and strangers from the deadly virus. The rare times people did venture outside their homes, they were understandably anxious and donned masks in the hope that this would mitigate its spread. Because of the risks of the virus, the outside world suddenly became dangerous in a way it had not been before the pandemic. Because we could not venture out, the world outside became continuous with the home: Rather than being the center of our lives and a refuge, for many of us it became our *whole* world. We let the world into our homes by working and learning at home. Our world became reduced to the microcosm of our homes while also becoming virtually continuous with the outside. For many people private and public became seamlessly connected, though only virtually. This seamless virtual world connecting our homes with people outside our homes became a "homescape."

But not everyone was so fortunate. Not everyone could avoid the dangers outside by reducing the world to the space of their homes thanks to various videoconferencing technologies such as Zoom, WebEx, and Google Meet. First, there were those who had to work outside the home, people who took care of the sick and dying in the hospitals or who sought to manage the influx of corpses from the hospital morgues—the "first responders." Another category of worker, those quickly dubbed "essential workers," assumed the risk of working outside their homes to provide goods and services to those safely confined to their homes. Restaurant workers, grocery workers, and delivery drivers quickly came to represent this new category of worker, likely because they were the ones who came to our homes to deliver us food or groceries, or, if we were either brave or foolish enough to venture out beyond the four walls of our refuge, these were the workers we encountered in the supermarkets and other stores that were able to remain open to the public.[2] Behind these workers we encountered through our masks were anonymous people most of us did not see and therefore did not think about, those who processed the meat and picked the produce we ate, and those who ensured that that these goods got to market on time.

The pandemic and its resulting lockdown also bred resentment among individuals who believed that the lockdown and various other regulations meant to control the spread of this deadly virus were but the latest example of state overreach. Conspiracies on social media fed the idea that the virus was not nearly as deadly as scientists and government authorities had claimed, that it was a mere diversion meant to mask the efforts by governments to control us. For these antigovernment conspiracy enthusiasts, this exercise of state power had to be resisted and the supposed hoax of the virus revealed. These individuals thought themselves imprisoned in their homes, their basic freedoms denied. I want to take seriously the belief by these antigovernment activists that they had become imprisoned in their homes in order to consider the possibility that their virulent opposition to stay-at-home orders was both a protest of state mandates and a protest against their identification as prisoners. This helps us to better see how anti-Black racism is central to their protests, since the incarcerated population is predominately nonwhite. By imprisoning people in their homes, the federal government was treating white people like those who were incarcerated, thereby denying them the privileges of whiteness. Here, I enlist the work of philosopher Charles Mills and his concept of "white ignorance" to make sense of the racial dimension of these lockdown protests in the United States during the spring and summer of 2020.

So I want to examine these three dimensions of how the meaning of "home" has changed during the pandemic: the blurring of the distinction between private realm of the home and the outside world that renders the home a quasi-public "homescape," the various assumptions that lie behind the distinction between nonessential and essential workers and what this distinction reveals about economic and racial inequality in the United States, and how racial resentment informed the understanding of home by individuals who protested against state-mandated lockdowns. These three dimensions are not exhaustive, but I believe they do begin to show some of the ways the meaning of "home" changed during this time of COVID that we are still enduring as I write this.

What I have called the "homescape" consists of a blurring of the public and private realms. In order to understand this, we must consider some salient political dimensions of home. The first section presents a brief account of neoliberalism. Neoliberalism is an ambiguous term with a number of different meanings, prompting some critics to claim that this ambiguity renders it meaningless. I acknowledge the ambiguity of the term, but I believe that properly understood, the term can be useful for helping us to understand the political stakes of the present.

In the second section I turn to recent accounts of home by author and theorist Toni Morrison and the account of the transformations of the public and private realm in neoliberalism by Bonnie Honig and Wendy Brown, two political theorists who use historical texts to illuminate the political situation of the present.

The third section on the figure of the essential worker draws upon the distinction between labor, work, and action as the three basic realms of human activity proposed by Hannah Arendt, while the final section on the white racial resentment fueling anti-lockdown protests is informed by the work of Mills. Arendt was a twentieth-century thinker who, like political theorists Honig and Brown, sought to make sense of the present. Arendt was motivated by ancient Greek thought to think through the demise of an autonomous political realm that could be distinguished from the necessities of life and the environments that we make ourselves. A Jewish émigré who fled Nazi totalitarianism for the United States, she also sought to make sense of totalitarianism. Mills, a contemporary political philosopher, diagnoses how white supremacy undergirds modern liberal political identity. He claims that the social contract that binds us together in a political community is underwritten by a racial contract that spells out the racist hierarchy that continues to structure society into the present.

COVID-19 AS A NEOLIBERAL CRISIS

To begin to make sense of these tangled senses of home, we need to consider various philosophical and political meanings of "home." This is not to deny that this word has many other important meanings, but I shall limit myself to these two in this chapter. Philosophical and political senses of home come into better focus once we acknowledge that homes have always been gendered and racialized spaces.

A couple examples will help clarify this claim. Consider the familiar phrase "A woman's place is in the home." Until recently, the assumption was that a household consisted of a married man and woman, and that the man would be the sole breadwinner while the woman took care of the household. Other domestic arrangements were considered abnormal and individuals in these arrangements were shunned. Women who did work outside the home typically found themselves in professions with less prestige and earning power, such as primary school teachers or nurses. These professions were once deemed "women's work." Furthermore, in popular culture these heteronormative families were portrayed as overwhelmingly white. Black women were expected to serve as housekeepers and nannies in middle- and upper-class white homes. This was considered the norm, and we need to keep this in mind to avoid the temptation of idealizing or romanticizing home life in the past.

Historically, policies governing the poor have encouraged this sort of family structure.[3] The Federal Housing Administration (FHA) insured home loans, thus encouraging home ownership. Melinda Cooper points out how the standard thirty-year mortgage backed by the FHA favored borrowers who were white and middle-class:

> The FHA imposed strict underwriting criteria on lenders, dictating everything from the acceptable payment structure of mortgages to housing models, location, and borrower profile, and banks needed to conform to these guidelines if they wished to receive federal guarantees. Ultimately it was the FHA that decided who was credit-worthy enough to receive a low-interest mortgage. The overall effect of such oversight was to restrict mortgage finance to the married, white man and exclude Fordism's non-normative subjects for the forms of wealth accumulation that flowed from home ownership in the post-war area.[4]

Cooper begins her book by claiming that "[t]he history of the family is one of perpetual crisis."[5] Theorists and policy makers on both the left and the right have attributed this crisis to one of "fatherlessness":

> Young, impoverished women, particularly African Americans and Latinas, are still having children out of wedlock and still expecting the welfare state to take care of them. In the 1990s, social theorists complicated this story somewhat when they announced that the long-standing, quasi-mythical crisis of the African American family, infamously diagnosed by the neoconservative Daniel Patrick Moynihan in 1965, had now spread to the white middle class, encouraging generations to forsake the stability of marriage in favor of career-minded narcissism.[6]

The Moynihan Report famously blamed a host of problems affecting the African American community on missing fathers and single mothers. In other words, it attributes social problems to the family, and by the 1980s this had become conventional wisdom, especially among conservatives in the United States. Consider the smear of the "welfare queen," which managed to be racist and misogynistic at the same time. Whether or not the family is indeed always in crisis, political commentators have a stake in making it seem in crisis. During COVID, political perception and reality appear to have coincided.

"Neoliberalism" is a term that defies easy definition, thanks in large part to the ambiguity mentioned previously. Nevertheless, Angela Davis nicely summarizes the meaning of the term when she writes that it indicates the shift, beginning in the 1980s, toward "an almost total freedom of movement for capital, goods, and services—in other words, the absolute rule of the market. Public expenditures for social services have been drastically cut. There has been constant pressure for the elimination of government intervention and regulation of the market."[7] Public services have been privatized, thus hollowing out the state. State power means promoting market capitalism, with individuals understood as agents of the market, who have value based solely upon their spending and earning power. Davis concludes that "neoliberalism sees the market as the very paradigm of freedom, and democracy emerges as a synonym for capitalism, which has reemerged as the telos of history."[8] In other words, capitalism comes to be understood as history's culmination, and societies that are governed by the rules and structures of the market rather than those of the state are preferable to those that rely upon a robust state with welfare programs such as universal healthcare, unemployment, and social security programs. In the United States, free-market fundamentalists call these state programs into question and criticize them for their alleged market inefficiencies.

COVID exposes the limitations of neoliberalism. Hollowed-out states cannot ensure the safety of their citizens during a pandemic. A pathological individualism that denies all accounts of the common good have become commonplace. In the next section, I consider how COVID lockdown transformed the home into a "homescape," a quasi-public space that is no longer private. The subsequent section shows how Arendt's conception of labor informs our designation of the "essential worker," the one who must labor outside the home to process the consumer goods that people need. The final section turns to a consideration of the racial dynamics of the lockdown protests.

COVID'S CHANGED HOMESCAPE: THE HOME AS VIRTUAL PUBLIC THING

In the introduction, I pointed to three possible ways that the meaning of home changed for people during COVID lockdown. Of course, this is not meant to be an exhaustive list, but I do believe these three aspects are significant and that we can make sense of them through philosophical reflection. For many of us, the intimate space of the home suddenly became a homescape: a site that was open to uninvited strangers who were now virtually in our home. Our coworkers and fellow students were now virtually part of our homes for much of the day. The private home became part of a homescape: a virtual classroom or office that was no longer exclusively private space. "Homescape" designates this changed space of the home, transformed from a private space into a virtual or quasi-public one. Television personalities were forced to broadcast their talk shows and news reports from their homes, and individuals on Twitter discussed which book titles they could detect on celebrities' shelves.[9] Ordinary people had unprecedented access to celebrities' homes, while everyone who suddenly found themselves working from home had to allow access to strangers in ways they never had before. But people's relationship to the outside world changed, too: Suddenly outdoors became a menacing space where the virus lurked. Political theorist Bonnie Honig wrote in 2017 about how Donald Trump's presidency signals the decline of what she calls "public things."[10] Drawing on a wide array of thinkers, including Hannah Arendt, D. W. Winnicott, and Jonathan Lear, she argues that the Trump presidency accelerated tendencies already found in neoliberalism toward the decline and eventual elimination of a freestanding public sphere or any shared notion of the common good. Neoliberalism is a form of government that strives for the privatization and economization of everything at the expense of all public things. Public things include the shared infrastructure that we easily forget about unless it fails. Honig cites the power grid, transportation infrastructure, and the sewer system as examples of public things.[11] These public things that grounded our shared civic identity have been increasingly privatized, and this is one of the central motifs of neoliberalism. Central to Honig's account of neoliberalism is this loss of public things and a shared sense of the common good; neoliberalism therefore is understood as an age of decline from a time when Americans identified with a common purpose and of the loss of these public things.

Does the crisis we are currently living through prompt us to rethink such narratives of decline and loss, and if so, how? It will take time to definitively answer this question, but there are signs that neoliberalism's influence may be waning. From the beginning of the pandemic in early 2020, many people claimed that the pandemic would accelerate trends of inequality already present in contemporary society, thereby updating the argument that Honig made in 2018, two years before the pandemic transformed so many lives. Quarantine as a response to pandemic demands isolation to an unprecedented degree, and this isolation that so many decry is a privilege only if we are fortunate to work in fields that permit us to isolate from others—that is, if we are not deemed "essential." Those of us deemed inessential are quarantined in our homes, while workers deemed "essential" are exposed to risks of illness and premature death to degrees not seen prior to the pandemic. What are the political stakes of COVID-19 and the collective response to it, including most prominently quarantine, and could it force us to rethink the political significance of the home, beyond an analysis that points to the economization of everything within the framework of neoliberalism? In other words, could COVID-19 and its crises help us to get past the limits of neoliberalism and its attendant slow-motion human and natural disasters?

In her own reflections on "home" from 2002, the fiction writer and essayist Toni Morrison points out that globalization threatens the "distortion of the public and the destruction of the private."[12] Unlike most theorists of neoliberalism, who conceive of neoliberal governmentality as an expansion of the private realm at the expense of public or common goods, Morrison points out that neoliberalism and globalization threaten the independence of both the private and public realms, or at least it threatens to fundamentally transform our experience of them. Explaining that globalism means the mass movement of people around the globe at levels not seen since the height of the slave trade in the eighteenth century, Morrison claims that most of this movement consists of people from former colonies to metropolitan centers for better jobs and refugees fleeing war-torn countries in the hope of better lives. Hence borders have become a focus of political debate in many countries.

We recall how Trump made the policing of borders a centerpiece of his 2016 presidential campaign. In 2020, as members of his administration finally began to grasp the threat posed by COVID-19, he sought to show that he had the virus under control by closing US borders and prohibiting travel from many European and Asian nations, thereby rendering Morrison's words prophetic. While Morrison understands the promise of globalization, she is more circumspect about its dangers than many commentators at the turn of the millennium, who tended to focus more on the promises of globalization than negative effects. Writing shortly after 9/11, she notes, "We glean what is public primarily, but not exclusively, from media. We are asked to abandon much of what was once private to the data-collecting requirements of government, political, and now security needs."[13] She sees that the divide between public and private had become more porous than ever, and she cites as examples the privatization of prisons and schools. Already, Morrison understands the dangers of what was to become social media, though in 2002 the concern with the media focus on private lives and government focus on private data were distinct concerns and not the urgent problem that social media would make them as companies like Facebook and Twitter encouraged people to make their lives more public while mining the data of their private lives. People had already become more open about their private lives, which fed the market for tabloids, talk shows, and reality television:

> There is private space (atriums, gardens, etc.) open to the public. And public spaces (parks, playgrounds, and beaches in certain neighborhoods) limited to private use. There is the looking-glass phenomenon of the "play" of the public in our private, interior lives. Interiors of our houses look like store displays (along with shelf after shelf of "collections") and store displays are arranged as house interiors; young people's behavior is said to be an echo of what the screen offers; the screen is said to echo, represent, youthful interests and behavior—not create them. Since the space in which both civic and private life has become so indistinguishable from inner and outer, from inside/outside, these two realms have been compressed into a ubiquitous blur, a rattling of our concept of home.[14]

We might recall Andy Warhol's quip about how everyone is entitled to their fifteen minutes of fame here, but Morrison reminds us to be careful. As our private lives become more public, our sense of privacy becomes eroded. Additionally, Morrison worries that with the erosion of the private self, individuals lose a sense of who they really are. Unlike political theorists Honig and Brown, who claim that neoliberalism leads to the withering of public things, Morrison sees our present age as one that transforms both our public and private lives in ways that help us better see how COVID-19 has changed our senses of home: The private realm assumes traits of the public at the same time that the public becomes more private.

Although Morrison wrote "The Foreigner's Home" just after 9/11 and therefore she could not have anticipated the rise of social media in the years after it was published, her essay anticipates its rise. On social media, everyone portrays themselves as if they were a star, and we live in a world of "social media influencers," individuals whose sole talent lies in their ability to generate clicks.[15] As Morrison saw, in a world where the private and public have come to permeate one another, it becomes much easier to become lost and not know exactly where one belongs: "To what do we pay greatest allegiance? Family, language group, culture, country, gender? Religion, race? And if none of these matter, are we urbane, cosmopolitan, or simply lonely? In other words, how do we decide where we belong? What convinces us that we do? Or put another way, what is the matter with foreignness?"[16] The problem is that home is a site of belonging, but as the space of home becomes confused with the public spaces outside it, then it becomes increasingly difficult to determine where exactly we belong. This feeling of alienation is heightened when the "place" where we spend much of our time is the virtual space of social media or on Zoom calls for work or school.

Still, we should avoid idealizing the meaning of home. "Home" has always been a fraught concept in which power dynamics that manifest themselves publicly in society as a whole play out in miniature in the home, despite the idyllic image of the home as a place of safety and refuge. As Matthew Desmond notes,

> Civic life too begins at home, allowing us to plant roots and take ownership over our community, participate in local politics, and reach out to neighbors in a spirit of solidarity and generosity. "It is difficult to force a man out of himself and get him to take an interest in the affairs of the whole state," Alexis de Tocqueville once observed. "But if it is a question of taking a road past his property, he sees at once that this small public matter has a bearing on his greatest private interests." It is only after we begin to see a street as *our* street, a public park as *our* park, a school as *our* school, that we can become engaged citizens, dedicating our time and resources for worthwhile causes: joining the Neighborhood Watch, volunteering to beautify a playground, or running for school board.[17]

Home provides us a sense of belonging not just to its intimate spaces but also to a broader civic life. While classical liberalism assumes a clear distinction between the public and private realms, this distinction was challenged as soon as it was proposed, and challenges to this founding distinction have continued down to the present. More recently, philosophers and political theorists have argued that neoliberalism means the market privatization of public, common goods. While I acknowledge that the surrender of public things to private corporations is happening, the claim that this is strictly due to privatization oversimplifies things. As Morrison notes, what we are actually witnessing is the transformation of the traditional distinction between the private realm of the home and the public social and political realm. Life under COVID during the past year makes these various transformations all the more apparent. While Desmond's hope that a firm sense of belonging that one finds securely in one's home will lead to a sense of civic belonging and shared political agency, Morrison's circumspection is certainly warranted.

HOME AS FREE SPACE: THE FIGURE OF THE ESSENTIAL WORKER AND THE PRIVILEGES OF HOME

Under lockdown, a previously unrecognized distinction suddenly became commonplace: the distinction between those who could work from home and were presumably "nonessential" (though it would certainly be rude to call them that!) and those who were deemed "essential." However, those workers confined to their homes (the "nonessential workers") were those who had the luxury of working from their homes, and their salaries typically reflected this privilege. The essential workers, by contrast, were individuals risking their health and indeed their lives often for a mere fraction of the salaries commanded by the more privileged lawyers, teachers, and businesspeople who were safe in their homes—people typically considered "white-collar" workers. Economic inequality has long been understood as a problem by politicians and theorists on the Left, but now this economic inequality had become immediately life threatening in a way it had not been before. Prior to COVID, the grind of those toiling in low-wage jobs led to a slow death; during COVID the immediate threat of death became an ever-present danger. Of course, race and class have long served as key predictors of longevity in the United States, a demographic fact that has led geographer Ruth Wilson Gilmore to define racism as "the state-sanctioned or extralegal production and exploitation of group-differentiated vulnerability to premature death."[18] Perhaps the pandemic made some people see this for the first time.

Home has always been both a lived and an imagined space. Saidiya Hartman captures the imagined dimension of home in her memoir *Lose Your Mother*:

> For the first and second generations born in captivity, the Americas were the only home they knew. Yet this did not stop them from dreaming of a province free of masters, plantations, whips, and the four degrees of torture. Even if Creoles could not share the ardor of their parents for the country lost, did they fancy it anyway? Or were imagined countries always doomed to be evanescent? Or did the opposite hold true: Were the only countries able to entice us and to grab hold of our hearts the ones we imagined?[19]

Hartman captures the melancholy yearning for home that her enslaved ancestors felt while she also questions whether "home" can ever be something more than an imaginary space for those captured in their African homes and enslaved in a country far from these ancestral homes. Indeed, Hartman continues, "it is only when you are stranded in a hostile country that you need a romance of origins; it only when you *lose your mother* that she becomes a myth; it is only when you fear the dislocation of the new that the old ways become precious, imperiled, and what your great-great-great-grandchildren one day wistfully describe as African."[20] Hartman's pressing question here concerns whether one can feel nostalgia for a home one has never known, a question that becomes more vexing when we as readers realize that the Ghana to which Hartman has returned in search of her ancestors bears little more than a passing resemblance to the home that, if it once existed, is now more an imagined landscape than it is a memory, if it can even be said to be a memory at all. More imagined than remembered, this home becomes all the more precious as a result.

Hartman's questions complicate the simple nostalgia for home as a space of security to which authors such as Matthew Desmond appeal. Desmond's project shows that this yearning for home as a space of safety is an ideal undercut by the reality of Melinda Cooper's family in crisis. Senator Moynihan's attribution of alleged Black racial pathologies to the crisis of the Black family complicates this yet further.

The latest chapter of this family crisis comes takes the form of the "essential worker," the worker whose job is to maintain the lives of those of us who are privileged enough to work from home during the pandemic. Furthermore, the figure of the "essential worker" extends Hannah Arendt's account of the home as a space of necessity, a space devoted to the necessary functions of life.

Arendt was not a theorist of neoliberalism, but her work has influenced a number of current thinkers who consider how free market capitalism has transformed the state beginning in the 1970s. One of the key reasons for Arendt's influence is that she wrote about the decline of an independent political realm during the modern period. Drawing on ancient Greek thought, she sees the political dimension of life as the realm of action, which she distinguishes from labor and work as the three main realms of human activity.

The reason my analysis of how our various understandings of "home" have been transformed under COVID focuses on Arendt's neo-Aristotelian account of the political conceptions of home is twofold: First, this Aristotelian account continues to be influential, with contemporary thinkers such as Wendy Brown and Bonnie Honig acknowledging their debt to her work. Additionally, I want to consider Arendt's accounts of home as the realm of the social because, despite their shortcomings, which will become more evident as we proceed, this Arendtian account demonstrates a clear connection between the home and necessity, a connection that will be important for us to see how the transformed conception of home relate to conceptions of home transformed as a result of the pandemic. Arendt reads Aristotle as advocating a political life of action in which citizens participate in the public life of their communities as a requirement for human flourishing. Without political participation, a flourishing life becomes a life merely lived. The essential worker is defined by the maintenance of mere life.

In her astute analysis of the philosophical and political stakes of neoliberalism, Brown draws on this distinction between a fulfilled life and mere life that Arendt also drew upon and that extends back to Aristotle. After claiming that a defining feature of contemporary society is the economization of all aspects of life, she writes,

> It is difficult to overstate the significance for democracy of these remakings of the purpose and orientations of both states and citizens. Of course, they entail the dramatic curtailment of public values, public goods, and popular participation in political life. They facilitate the increasing power of large corporations to fashion law and policy for their own ends, not simply crowding out, but overtly demoting the public interest. Obviously, too, governance according to market metrics displaces classic liberal democratic concerns with justice and balancing diverse interests. As economic parameters become the only parameters for all conduct and concern, the limited form of human existence that Aristotle and later Hannah Arendt designated as "mere life" and that Marx called life "confined by necessity"—concern with survival and wealth acquisition—this limited form and imaginary becomes ubiquitous and total *across* classes.[21]

In other words, one of the main features of neoliberalism as Brown (and, following her, Honig and other political theorists) understands it is that neoliberalism is a form of life in which life can be understood only in economic terms. Of course, *oikos*, the Greek root of English words such as "economics" and "ecology," means "home." So neoliberalism reconfigures life strictly in terms of home, albeit home understood in a particular way: as the realm of necessity, a domain governed by the patriarch where free political action has no place.

In ancient Greece, this household space was structured as such a patriarchal space. The male head of the household (*kyrios*) dominated the other members of the household and was responsible for all the dependents in the home, which could include his wife, his children, and his slaves. Free action for male citizens in democratic city-states such as Athens was possible in the public sphere, while the home was the realm of the family, and he was its head. With some variations, this patriarchal model of home and family persists throughout much of history. One of the key innovations of modernity is that this intimate space of the home becomes structured in terms of both patriarchal and racial domination. With the advent of chattel slavery and the racist ideology that supported it, it became necessary to qualify that this household head was both white and male.[22] No doubt there were exceptions to this even in the years prior to the American Civil War, but nevertheless the model household was headed by a white man. Although my account here is condensed, it serves to remind us of the legacies of the home as a patriarchal and racialized space, and these legacies are important to keep in mind as we consider how this pandemic has changed the various senses of "home."

In addition to its figuration first as a patriarchal and later as a racially stratified space, the *oikos* has been understood by thinkers such as Aristotle and Arendt as a space of necessity. Lacking in political significance, the home is a realm of tasks necessary solely for the maintenance of life. The home is the space where we carry out bodily tasks such as sleeping, eating, and sex. Hence Aristotle claims that the *oikos* lacks political significance, for politics is the public space of agency and free action, a space in which only men could appear. When contemporary political theorists such as Brown and Honig lament the loss of this public sphere, what they typically lament is the modern version of Aristotle's public sphere.

Arendt is the political theorist who has done the most to provide a modern account of Aristotle's political realm and his attempt to distinguish it from the prepolitical realm of necessity, so given their concerns it makes sense that both Brown and Honig have been influenced by Arendt's writing. The most concise account of these essential human realms of labor work and action occurs in *The Human Condition* and her summary in "Labor, Work, Action."

"Labor, Work, Action" was originally a 1964 lecture delivered at the University of Chicago's Divinity School as part of a conference with the theme of "Christianity and Economic Man: Moral Decisions in an Affluent Society."[23] This context is important, because in this lecture Arendt reiterates her critique of various Marxist attempts to render politics solely in economic terms. She begins by asking what we mean by action, and then restates the classic distinction between a *vita contemplativa* and a *vita active*, a life devoted to contemplation and one devoted to action. While Arendt acknowledges the priority that religion and philosophy traditionally accorded the contemplative life, she argues that various activities provide the conditions for a contemplative life and hence should be considered primary.[24] This distinction between a contemplative life and one devoted to labor is also the basis for the distinction between essential and nonessential workers (which we discuss more fully below):

> Traditionally therefore the *vita activa* received its meaning from the *vita contemplativa;* a very restricted dignity was bestowed upon it because it served the needs and wants of contemplation in a living body. Christianity with its belief in a hereafter, whose joys announce themselves in the delights of contemplation, conferred a religious sanction upon the abasement of the *vita active* while, on the other hand, the command to love your neighbor acted as a counterweight against this estimation unknown to antiquity.[25]

Arendt traces a key shift in the modern period from the prioritization of work to labor as the highest human activity. Whereas the ancient Greeks had prized work, moderns prized labor. Action is the activity associated with politics, labor is the necessary activity we undertake in order to maintain our lives, and work is the activity of the craftsperson that results in a tangible handmade product. Labor produces consumer goods instead of a finished work of craft or art: "Labor in other words produces consumer goods, and laboring and consumer goods, and laboring and consuming are but two stages of the ever-recurring cycle of biological life."[26] Labor puts people in an endless cycle of activity that produces goods to be consumed so that more goods can be produced. There is nothing durable about consumer goods; our world was once composed of the products of work, activity that produces a durable artifact that we can use or contemplate. On the other hand, labor is tied to the biological process: "Labor, caught in the cyclical movement of the biological process, has neither a beginning nor an end properly speaking—only pauses, intervals between exhaustion and regeneration."[27]

Essential labor is the labor of necessity. Examples include food delivery, restaurant work, and meatpacking. Prior to the pandemic, these typically low-skill, low-wage positions were filled by members of marginalized groups, such as immigrants and minorities. COVID made these jobs far more deadly and hence less desirable than they had been previously. Stories abound of owners unable to staff their restaurants and schools unable to staff support positions. It seems that people are deciding that the risks of doing these jobs outweigh the benefits and that they are better off staying home.

Conservative politicians in many states are trying to deny extended unemployment benefits in the hopes that essential workers will be forced back to work—that is, forced back into the precarious jobs burdened with risks that well-off politicians and other members of the elite need not face. The burdens of COVID fall disproportionately on poor people and communities of color. In this respect, COVID is nothing new, but the hope is that this might lead to real political change in the United States.

THE WHITE IGNORANCE OF THE CONFINED AND PRIVILEGED

Racial and economic inequalities can be found in the work that people do and the jobs that are available to them. But there are certainly other ways that racism has become manifest during COVID. In this section, I want to look at some possible motivations for the backlash against the quarantine measures among those individuals, predominantly conservatives in the United States, who protested against the lockdown measures and the conception of home or the expanded homescape that informed these demonstrations. Specifically, I want to consider how the sense that they had been trapped or imprisoned in their homes motivated at least some people to protest COVID restrictions imposed by various states and the federal government in the United States. Due to the realities of the carceral state and the racial inequalities inherent punishment in the United States, the protests were at least in some cases informed by racial resentments.

Indeed, in an essay written for *Vox* in April 2020, Maia Niguel Hoskin connects antilockdown protests with white privilege.[28] She reports that protestors in Michigan, Washington, Maryland, and Texas marched with signs declaring "Live Free or Die" and many protestors were armed with automatic rifles, and she recalls the storming of the Wisconsin state capitol on April 23, 2020, in which protestors condemning Governor Tom Eyers's "Safer at Home" lockdown measures that had been recently extended until May 26.[29] Some commentators have argued that these antilockdown protests were a rehearsal for the violent riots at the US Capitol in Washington, DC, on January 6, 2021.[30]

These well-armed protesters were permitted to demonstrate unmolested by authorities. This is in marked contrast to many of the protests responding to the deaths of George Floyd and Breonna Taylor in the summer of 2020. While many of these protests were peaceful, there were notable clashes with police in cities such as New York, Portland, and Washington, DC. CNN reported that Washington, DC, police arrested five times more people during the height of the George Floyd protests during the summer of 2020 than they did during the Capitol riots of January 6: "The District's police made 61 'unrest-related' arrests on Wednesday, compared with 316 on June 1, when protesters and rioters filled city streets a week after Minneapolis police killed George Floyd. That was the same day as Trump's infamous Bible-holding photo op, when law enforcement officers dispersed mostly peaceful protesters with tear gas."[31]

Racism was likely a factor here, though this is often disavowed by pundits and politicians alike, especially conservative ones. Philosopher Charles Mills provides conceptual tools for thinking through the widespread denial of racism, particularly among white people in the United States.

Mills traces an implicit racial contract that underlies the explicit social contract forming the basis of society. This racial contract is a tacit expression of white supremacy. As Mills writes at the outset of *The Racial Contract,* it "is the unnamed political system that made the modern world what it is today."[32] His task is to make explicit this political system that he names the racial contract. This political contract has three different dimensions: It is simultaneously moral, political, and epistemological.[33] This racial contract is historical and accounts for the denial and historical amnesia around racism today: "One could say then, as a general rule, that *white misunderstanding, misrepresentation, evasion, and self-deception on matters related to race* are among the most pervasive mental phenomena of the past few hundred years, a cognitive and moral economy psychically required for conquest, colonization, and enslavement."[34] The racial contract underwrites the political and moral order of white supremacy that justifies conquest, colonization, and enslavement. While we may comfort ourselves by saying that slavery and colonization have been abolished, paeans to racial progress and enlightenment ignore the new forms that colonization and slavery take in our allegedly "postracial" society.

The political dimension provides an account of the origins of society. The classic contract theorists of the seventeenth and eighteenth centuries posited a state of nature prior to society or government. In the twentieth century, their successor John Rawls asks us to imagine what sort of society we would devise if we did not know what our position in society would be, whether we would be rich or poor, Black or white, or a man or woman. Mills defines this racial contract as "that set of formal or informal agreements" among people who conceive of themselves as white as full persons while designating those who are not deemed white as "of a different and inferior moral status."[35] Members of the police, military, and penal system enforce this racial contract, and this helps explain the disparate arrest records of Black Lives Matter protestors and 1/6 protestors: "The coercive arm of the state, then—the police, the penal system, the army—need to be seen as in part the enforcers *of* the Racial Contract, working both to keep the peace and prevent crime among the white citizens, and to maintain the racial order and detect and destroy challenges to it so that across the white settler state nonwhites are incarcerated at different rates and for longer terms."[36] The resentment that drives antilockdown protests and the 1/6 protest stems from the sense that this implicit white supremacist hierarchy is endangered. There are euphemisms for "white supremacy," such as "traditional way of life" or "white working class," but the danger that white protestors see is one that undermines this hierarchy. The police and military serve as protectors of this hierarchy, so their authority cannot be undermined without also undermining the white supremacist hierarchy of the racial contract.

Mills begins "White Ignorance" by observing that epistemology, and by implication philosophy itself, begins by universalizing from a particular cultural experience of knowledge and ignorance that can be summarized as the Cartesian moment. Descartes sought to avoid error at all costs by discovering or erecting stout conceptual bulwarks against it, a task the American philosopher John Dewey has aptly called "the quest for certainty." This Cartesian quest for certainty and the epistemology it has engendered assumes the standpoint of the solitary individual who can distinguish truth from falsity through effort. Neglected is the role that society plays in the formation of knowledge. According to Mills, the biases that initially blinded epistemologists to the fundamental role society plays in truth formation were eventually rectified during the 1960s in the American context by thinkers such as W. V. O. Quine, who were building upon insights borrowed from pragmatists such as William James and John Dewey. However, even in the post-Quinean era, the social world that epistemologists investigated was one that assumed only white male members. In other words, it was colorblind in the same facile way that people claim "to not see race" today: It was blind to the pervasive ways that racial thinking still colors how we see and what we think, even if we are not consciously aware of it. In short, white ignorance precisely ignores the various effects that the racial ordering of society based upon white supremacist principles had in the past and the manifold ways that this racist ordering of society continues to affect how we see and think of ourselves in the present. Mills summarizes his argument thusly:

> White ignorance has been able to flourish all these years because a white epistemology of ignorance has safeguarded it against the dangers of an illuminating Blackness or redness, protecting those who for "racial" reasons have needed not to know. Only by starting to break these rules and meta-rules can we begin the long process that will lead to the eventual overcoming of this white darkness and the achievement of an enlightenment that is genuinely multiracial.[37]

In addition to the failure to see the epistemic commitments of white supremacy, for Mills white ignorance entails that individuals accept a positive mythology of whiteness. Mills makes the case for white myth-making as an aspect of white ignorance; that is, white identity requires the one see oneself as innocent and free.

White innocence firmly secures these assumptions against the evidence of reality and thereby makes it possible to either ignore how one's ancestors violently subjugated people belonging to so-called lesser races (white ignorance) or it serves to justify such subjugation of people in the past (white mythologizing). Furthermore, one is unable to comprehend that such practices extend into the present.

The anxiety underlying these antilockdown protests can be better understood if we keep the conceptual framework of the racial contract in mind. White racial resentment fueled the protests in Charlottesville and other protests during the Trump presidency. The anxiety that is sometimes overtly expressed ("Jews will not replace us!") but more often implied in these protests is the anxiety that the white supremacist racial order is waning. Protesters' refusal of imprisonment in their homes is a rejection of being identified with members of a racial and economic underclass subject to incarceration and heightened police surveillance. Home becomes something akin to imprisonment here. White protesters' secure place at the top of the racial hierarchy is threatened, and this threat is implicit in their protests.

In this chapter, I have sought to survey some of the permutations of the meaning of "home" as a result of COVID. COVID makes apparent the various crises of a neoliberal political order in which individual states that have been hollowed out by forces of deregulation and privatization struggle to respond to a crisis that demands a collective response. Whether we will heed the lessons of COVID and face other challenges such as climate change or economic inequality collectively remains to be seen. Indeed, as I write this, it remains to be seen whether ignorance and individualism will make it impossible to face the ongoing challenges of COVID itself.

NOTES

1. Matthew Desmond, *Evicted* (New York: Penguin Random House, 2016), 368.
2. As I write this, the United States is in the midst of what economist Robert Reich has called an "apolitical general strike." While systematic data is currently lacking, at least anecdotally it seems that one of the contributing factors is that "essential workers" are thinking twice about whether they want to risk their lives for low wages during a pandemic. See Matt Cannon, "Robert Reich: American Workers are on Strike over Low Wage S*** Jobs," *Newsweek*, October 11, 2021, accessed October 17, 2021, https://www.newsweek.com/robert-reich-american-workers-strike-low-wage-jobs-employment-1637543.

3. Melinda Cooper provides a history of these policies in her book *Family Values: Between Neoliberalism and the New Social Conservatism* (New York: Zone Books, 2017). In it, she examines how neoliberalism and neoconservatism coordinate family policies in the United States in a way that focuses on personal responsibility and work.

4. Cooper, *Family Values*, 144–45.

5. Cooper, *Family Values*, 7.

6. Cooper, *Family Values*, 7.

7. Angela Davis, "Recognizing Racism in the Era of Neoliberalism" (2008), in *The Meaning of Freedom and Other Difficult Dialogues* (San Francisco: City Lights Books, 2012), 168.

8. Davis, "Recognizing Racism in the Era of Neoliberalism," 169.

9. Here is but one example of many: *Town and Country* magazine asked a celebrity book curator to judge the books on various celebrities' bookshelves. Olivia Hosken, "What a Celebrity Book Curator Really Thinks of A-Listers' Bookshelves," *Town and Country*, May 19, 2020, accessed April 12, 2021, https://www.townandcountrymag.com/style/home-decor/g32449315/zoom-bookshelves-ranked-books-style/

10. Bonnie Honig, *Public Things: Democracy and Disrepair* (New York: Fordham University Press, 2017).

11. Honig, *Public Things*, 3.

12. Toni Morrison, "The Foreigner's Home," in *The Source of Self-Regard: Selected Essays, Speeches and Meditations* (New York: Alfred A. Knopf, 2019), 7. This essay was originally presented as the Alexander Lecture at the University of Toronto in May 2002.

13. Morrison, "The Foreigner's Home," 7.

14. Morrison, "The Foreigner's Home," 7–8.

15. Bernard Harcourt reflects on the rise of social media in terms of the possibilities and dangers of what he terms "the expository society" in his book *Exposed: Desire and Disobedience in the Digital Age* (Cambridge, MA: Harvard University Press, 2015). Harcourt traces the manifold ways that our online lives are subject to both government scrutiny as well as the scrutiny of private corporations such as Facebook and Amazon. He opens with this reminder: "Every routine act on our iPads and tablets, on our laptops, notebooks, and Kindles, office PCs and smartphones, every transaction with our debit card, gym pass, E-Z Pass bus pass and loyalty cards can be archived, data-mined, and traced back to us. Linked together or analyzed separately, these data points constitute a new virtual identity, a digital self that is now more tangible, authoritative, and demonstrable, more fixed and provable than our analog selves" (1).

16. Harcourt, *Exposed*, 8.

17. Desmond, *Evicted*, 368–69.

18. Ruth Wilson Gilmore, *Golden Gulag: Prisons, Surplus, Crisis, and Opposition in Globalizing California* (Berkley: University of California Press, 2007), 28.

19. Saidiya Hartman, *Lose Your Mother: A Journey along the Atlantic Slave Route* (New York: Farrar, Straus and Giroux, 2007), 98.

20. Hartman, *Lose Your Mother*, 98.

21. Wendy Brown, *Undoing the Demos: Neoliberalism's Stealth Revolution* (New York: Zone Books, 2015), 43.

22. Recent scholarship has begun to complicate this simple picture, however. For good recent examples of scholarship that complicate it, see Stephanie Jones-Rogers, *They Were Her Property: White Women as Property Owners in the American South* (New Haven, CT: Yale University Press, 2019), and Tommy J. Curry, *The Man-Not: Race, Class, Genre, and the Dilemmas of Black Manhood* (Philadelphia: Temple University Press, 2017). While Jones-Rogers focuses on white women slave owners, Curry reconsiders the scholarly account of Black masculinity found in white feminist thought.

23. Hannah Arendt, "Labor, Work, Action," in *The Portable Hannah Arendt*, ed. Peter Baehr (New York: Penguin Books, 2000), 167.

24. Arendt, "Labor, Work, Action," 167.

25. Arendt, "Labor, Work, Action," 168.

26. Arendt, "Labor, Work, Action," 171.

27. Arendt, "Labor, Work, Action," 175.

28. Maia Niguel Hoskin, "The Whiteness of Anti-Lockdown Protests: How Ignorance, Privilege, and Anti-Black Racism Is Driving White Protestors to Risk Their Lives," *Vox*, April 25, 2020, accessed April 22, 2021, https://www.vox.com/first-person/2020/4/25/21234774/coronavirus-covid-19-protest-anti-lockdown.

29. Reid J. Epstein and Kay Nolan, "A Few Thousand Protest Stay-At-Home Order at Wisconsin State Capitol," *New York Times*, April 24, 2020, accessed April 22, 2021, https://www.nytimes.com/2020/04/24/us/politics/coronavirus-protests-madison-wisconsin.html.

30. See, e.g., Derek Hawkins and Kim Bellware, "After Trial Runs at State Houses Last Year, the Far Right's Violent Tactics Erupted at the Capitol," *Washington Post*, January 9, 2021, accessed September 13, 2021, https://www.washingtonpost.com/national-security/2021/01/09/capitol-riots-extremists/.

31. Casey Tolan, "DC Police Made Far More Arrests at the Height of Black Lives Matter Protests Than during the Capitol Clash," *CNN*, January 9, 2021, accessed September 13, 2021, https://www.cnn.com/2021/01/08/us/dc-police-arrests-blm-capitol-insurrection-invs/index.html.

32. Charles Mills, *The Racial Contract* (Ithaca, NY: Cornell University Press, 1997), 1.

33. Mills, *The Racial Contract*, 9.

34. Mills, *The Racial Contract*, 19.

35. Mills, *The Racial Contract*, 11.

36. Mills, *The Racial Contract*, 84.

37. Charles Mills, "White Ignorance," *Race and Epistemologies of Ignorance*. Ed. Shannon Sullivan and Nancy Tuana (New York: State University of New York Press, 2007), 35.

Chapter 3

Waiting to Say Goodbye

J. S. Biehl[1]

"Michael O'Sullivan was my great friend, but I don't ever remember telling him that." So begins the character Jackie O'Shea's touching and tender funeral oration in the 1998 film *Waking Ned Devine*. His moving speech takes place against the farcical backdrop that defines the movie itself. Michael O'Sullivan is not dead but is rather among those gathered to pay their respects. The funeral is for Ned Devine, who died suddenly from shock upon learning that he had won millions in the lottery. Pained at the thought of such good fortune going to waste, the residents of the fictious remote Irish town scheme to convince the authorities that Ned is still alive, with the aim of dividing the winnings among themselves. As he is about to eulogize Ned, the lottery agent investigating the claim enters the church, forcing Jackie to improvise. He continues:

> The words that are spoken at a funeral are spoken too late for the man that is dead. What a wonderful thing it would be to visit your own funeral. To sit at the front and hear what was said. Maybe to say a few things yourself. Michael and I grew old together. But at times, when we laughed, we grew younger. If he was here now, if he could hear what I say, I'd congratulate him on being a great man. And thank him for being a friend.

I have seen this scene several times now, as watching the film has become something of a St. Patrick's Day tradition among my family. Yet it was clear to all of us that the circumstances of our viewing on March 17, 2020, were different. Indeed, the circumstances of everything were different. A week earlier, on the 11th, the school where I teach announced we would be moving to remote instruction for the remainder of the semester. My wife's office closed indefinitely on the 13th. On Sunday the 15th, Mayor Bill DeBlasio did what seemed simultaneously unthinkable and inevitable and announced the shuttering of the New York City public school system, rendering my three sons—and more than a million other children besides—homebound students for the foreseeable future. Then, on the following Sunday, March 22, Governor Andrew Cuomo essentially closed New York State for anything beyond "essential" business.

Essential business included those working in shipping, media, warehousing, grocery and food production, pharmacies, utilities, banks and related financial institutions, and, of course, healthcare. It also included, as it always does, the work of dealing with death and dying. The dead keep coming, and during the height of the pandemic they were coming quickly. All of these industries and business sectors were affected by the pandemic and our response to it, but our business with death most profoundly. Wakes, memorial services, funerals, and attended burials could be held only if restricted to immediate family members, a restriction that in many instances had the consequence that such rituals were not being held at all.

During the remainder of March, and throughout a dreamlike but all-too-deadly April, I repeatedly encountered stories of brokenhearted families and friends unable to gather to mourn and remember loved ones. And whether they were in New York, in Seattle, or in the Italian city of Bergamo, the laments were the same. "For us, it's a trauma, an emotional trauma," said Alberto Ceresoli, the editor of a paper in Bergamo whose pages were swelling with the names of the recently deceased. "These are people who die alone and who are buried alone. They didn't have someone hold their hand and the funerals have to be tiny, with a quick prayer from the priest. Many of the close relatives are in quarantine."[2] "We can't properly bury our dead because of the situation," acknowledged Meri Dreyfuss of San Francisco, whose sister Barbara had died in Seattle. Meri was resigned to delaying any funeral because the virus and the resulting restrictions meant that "we can't mourn together, we can't share memories together, we can't get together and hug each other."[3]

I and people that I love have been touched by these tragic circumstances as well. My mother's best friend—a woman who, along with her family, was a fixture in my life, present at every holiday and celebration—died in April 2020. There was no funeral, no memorial service. Neither my mother nor I and my siblings could "say goodbye" to someone we loved and was so much a part of our lives. Much worse, this woman's children, dispersed across the country, could not come together to mourn and bury their mother and their children's grandmother. And because they could not be together, they could not provide themselves with the only form of comfort adequate to their grief: to cry in the arms of those who are grieving with you. Like love, grief manifests itself physically, and we instinctively seek contact with others who feel the same. The empathetic embrace of another often helps steady us in the midst of the breaking waves of emotion stirred up by that the death of those we love. Unable to communicate our grief in this urgent, visceral, and cathartic way, we risk being left adrift, suspended somewhere between our lives before our loss, when the person was a familiar presence, and our lives going forward, when we have become reconciled to living with only their memory. Having to navigate this journey from the one to the other alone, as my friends and so many others have been forced to do, is a lonely and bleak endeavor.

Nor, of course, is this whole extent of our current tragedy—the emotional ravages of the pandemic have not been limited to surviving friends and family, as those who from age or infirmity had already reason to reckon with their impending death were now forced to think of having to face it alone. The author of an article on what this was doing to New York City's elderly population warned that the psychological suffering wrought by the fear of dying alone amounted to "a second epidemic," and worried that "for many, it will do more harm than the virus itself."[4] I believe that both the fear of dying without the company of those we care most intimately about and the heartache of being unable to feel the solace of shared grief over the loss of those we have loved are central features of "a second epidemic" that is causing immeasurable harm. While COVID-19, the disease caused by the SARS-CoV-2 virus, threatens our biological welfare (at the time of writing—early October 2021—the World Health Organization estimates 5 million COVID-19 related deaths worldwide), some of the measures that we have taken to mitigate that threat, measures designed to spare human life, have imperiled features of our lives that are fundamental to making them uniquely human.

Defining what it is to be human seems to be humanity's perpetual business, yet Aristotle's effort to distinguish us from "beasts" and "gods" has managed to retain much of its influence over the course of more than two millennia, and I believe for good reason. In characterizing us as "political animals,"[5] Aristotle identified us as beings unable to sustain ourselves outside of the society of others, whether in the biologically immediate association of the family, or in the community that nature ultimately intends, the "state." But as significant as this denial of our self-sufficiency is, it is the capacity that Aristotle claims makes human society possible—namely, "the gift of speech"—on which so much of our self-understanding seems to depend. We come to appreciate the consequential nature of this endowment when he tells us that

> whereas mere voice is but an indication of pleasure or pain, and is therefore found in other animals . . . the power of speech is intended to set forth the expedient and inexpedient, and therefore likewise the just and the unjust. And it is a characteristic of man that he alone has any sense of good and evil, of just and

> unjust, and the like, and the association of living beings who have this sense makes a family and a state.[6]

To have a "sense of good and evil, just and unjust, and the like" is to exist not simply in the physical world that sustains the biological journey from birth to death of all living things, but to partake in a specifically human world that allows for and sustains our particular identities. It is only by virtue of being seen as recognizably unique individuals, rather than replaceable members of a species, that moral notions concerning how we treat one another have any point. "The power of speech" can "set forth the expedient and inexpedient, and therefore likewise the just and the unjust," only because it allows one to communicate *who I am*. Only creatures capable of answering (and asking) that question can be said to have not only pleasures and pains (and wants and needs) but also plans, projects, hopes, and values. While nonhuman animals often bond, and clearly grieve over the death of a mate or offspring, it seems the sole privilege of humans to recognize it as fitting, appropriate, and perhaps even a duty to honor, as Jackie did with Michael, another as a great person and to thank him or her for being a friend.

This world in which we can become peculiarly human—where we become *persons*, indeed, the irreplaceable person that each one of us cannot otherwise be—is not one we are born into or can possibly enter alone. With birth begins a life that requires nourishment and protection from dangers and disease to be sustained; becoming human, however, will require more. Without forming attachments to others who provide care and love, infants and young children face uncertain prospects for their emotional and social development.[7] Such attachments are the basis for the child's first formative relationships, formative because each such relationship amounts to a communal engagement that contributes to the formation of a unique and unprecedented individual who will eventually be capable of (hopefully peaceful and productive) social interaction with others he or she does not know.

These relationships begin, of course, with the "mothering" one provided by a principal caregiver (who often is though needn't always be the biological mother) for the child. While mothering is crucial for many animals, especially among mammals, human mothering is, as the philosopher Virginia Held observes, nevertheless a fundamentally "different activity from the mothering engaged in by other animals." Putting a finer point on Aristotle's definition of humans as political animals, Held describes how the distinctively human version of mothering makes such animals possible:

> Human mothering shapes language and culture, and forms human social personhood. Human mothering develops morality, it does not merely transmit techniques of survival; impressive as the latter can be, they do not have built into

> them the aims of morality. Human mothering teaches consideration for others based on moral concern; it does not merely follow and bring the child to follow instinctive tendency. Human mothering creates autonomous persons; it does not merely propagate a species. It can be fully as creative an activity as most other human activities; to create *new* persons, and new types of *persons*, is surely as creative as to make new objects, products, or institutions.[8]

And without in any sense diminishing the fundamental importance of the mothering role, we can add that the creation of new, autonomous persons, and new types of such persons, extends beyond childhood; it is the unending work of a lifetime and depends on the love, care, concern, and influence of many other persons, including other family members and ultimately, and very significantly, friends. With each new emotionally dependent interconnection we make with another we continue, in a new direction, our process of becoming who we are. No relationship based on reciprocated feelings (rather than, say, contingently applicable social roles) can fail to leave a person unchanged—for better or for worse—for having been a part of it. Our sense of self, of propriety, of what we owe to others, what others owe to us, and how much we expect those obligations to be met and by whom—what amounts to our moral nature (and the foundation of what Aristotle referred to as our sense of good and evil, and of just in unjust)—are all the product of the essential mutuality of the human condition.

Our prospects for a good life (and, indeed, our very ideas of what a good life might possibly be), depend greatly on our being willing and able to share our lives with and to share in the lives of others. More simply, for most people, a good life is not possible when pursued alone. To remind ourselves of this, to acknowledge that to live a life worth living is possible only through our emotionally intimate involvement with others, makes plain why so many of us cannot imagine that dying alone could possibly make for a good death. As an ineliminable feature of life, we generally think of and take the measure of death using the same notions and standards we apply to our lives. We want our deaths to be "meaningful" and to be "worthy" of the lives we have strived to lead. The thought of dying in fear, or in shame, or in loneliness is no less troubling to us than the prospect of living in such conditions. That we take ourselves to have far less control over how we die—and over whether it meets our own standards of a good death—than over how we live is, I believe, why contemplating our own deaths is so discomfiting. What is so frightening about the pandemic is that we recognize its ability to leave so many of us with no control over our deaths at all.

And so it is not at all an exaggeration to characterize the expectation of something so dire as dying alone as "a second epidemic" that for "many . . . will do more harm than the virus itself." Nor does it seem to be hyperbole to think of being denied that which we find most essential for a life worth living as being subject to a fate worse than death. To recoil from a life that cannot be measured in terms more compelling than mere biological survival is to condemn a death that amounts to no more than its mere cessation. We want our deaths to be as human as our lives: rooted in love, friendship, and ritual. Recognizing all of this is necessary for any remotely adequate appreciation for the magnitude of the dual tragedies resulting from the spread of the coronavirus and from our efforts to evade it. That we imposed (and in some cases continue to impose) such restrictions on hospital and nursing home visitations, for example, was no less devastating for being defensible. We assuredly saved lives through our draconian measures, yet we undoubtedly damaged others when we made it impossible for hands to be held, I love yous to be said, eulogies to be given, and glasses to be raised.

None of this is to say that we should not have reacted to the virus in the ways that we have. If we were risking only our own lives by keeping vigil at the bedsides of our loved ones, then I believe we would have overwhelming reason for criticism and complaint. But the risk could not (and still cannot) be reliably contained, and so the case for prioritizing survival over emotional comfort has seemed not simply pragmatically compelling, but morally so. Recognizing this, however, does not make it more appealing; it only heightens the tragic nature of our predicament. And while we have rightly honored "frontline" and "essential" workers for the heroic sacrifices they have made on our behalf, we should not forget those who have borne the burden of our mitigation strategies, forsaking goodbyes to those they have lost to protect the rest of us from the suffering the same heartbreaking tragedy. And I would thus beg restraint from those who seem eager to condemn them for harboring any resentment. A more compassionate response to their sacrifice is to become companions in remembrance. The *New York Times* "Those We've Lost" series aims "to convey the human toll of COVID-19 by putting faces and names to the growing numbers of the dead, and to portray them in all of their variety."[9] Focusing on the impact of the coronavirus in New York City, the online news outlet *The City*'s "Missing Them: Remembering the New Yorkers We've Lost to COVID-19" likewise seeks to restore our humanity in the face of death, by committing "to remember and honor every person who died—who they were and what they meant to this city."[10]

These welcome efforts serve to amplify (and in many cases to replace entirely) attempts through funerals and memorials to dignify the death of those we have lost by commending the lives they have lived. Yet it remains inescapably true, as Jackie O'Shea observed, "that the words that are spoken at a funeral are spoken too late for the man that is dead." Of course they are, but this unfortunate truth does not diminish the value of speaking them. Our rituals of remembrance, including our traditions of "waking" the dead, seem in part an attempt to escape the limitations of our own mortality, to assure ourselves that we will persist in the memories of the living and that they will continue to speak our names after we have departed from the world. This small measure of immortality is by no means insignificant, for it amounts to the honor we are each due for the lives that our love and friendship helped to shape and sustain.

There is another reason why the words spoken at a funeral matter so much, a reason many of us are at once grateful for and pained to acknowledge. The gatherings where we honor the memory of one who has died often prompt us to finally speak the words we wish we had spoken sooner. That someone is our great friend; that their love and happiness have been so central to our own; that we are grateful for the care, support, and attention that they have given us and for the faith they had in us that was at crucial moments greater than the faith we had in ourselves—these are things that many of us find difficult or embarrassing to say and assuage our self-disappointment by assuring ourselves that such sentiments are already well understood. And no doubt in many cases they are. Our humanity is rooted in our capacity for momentous speech and yet our natures often conspire to leave the most meaningful words we could say regrettably unsaid when they could do the most good.

It is part of the moral tragedy of the pandemic that we are losing opportunities to make amends by turning those words into a public testament to the importance of the person we have lost. Perhaps the only worthwhile response to this tragedy, therefore, is to commit to saying the things we want to say when we have the opportunities to say them. This will not prevent, undo, or ameliorate the wounds this pandemic is inflicting on our humanity; it will not change the calculus that results in people dying in emotional isolation, nor will it allow survivors to gather to comfort one another and to honor the memories of those who have passed. But it would be a humane thing to do in any case.

NOTES

1. This essay is dedicated to the memory of Nuala Brown

2. Jason Horowitz and Emma Bubola, "Italy's Coronavirus Victims Face Death Alone, with Funerals Postponed," *New York Times*, March 16, 2020, https://www.nytimes.com/2020/03/16/world/europe/italy-coronavirus-funerals.html.

3. Kirk Johnson, "Coronavirus Means Funerals Must Wait: 'We Can't Properly Bury Our Dead,'" *New York Times*, March 25, 2020, https://www.nytimes.com/2020/03/25/us/coronavirus-funerals.html.

4. John Leland, "At 89, She Fears Dying Alone More Than the Coronavirus Itself," *New York Times*, April 7, 2020, https://www.nytimes.com/2020/04/07/nyregion/dying-alone-coronavirus.html.

5. Aristotle, *Politics,* trans. Benjamin Jowett, in *The Basic Works of Aristotle*, ed. Richard McKeon (New York: Random House, 1941), (1253a 7 –10).

6. Aristotle, *Politics*, trans. Benjamin Jowett, in *The Basic Works of Aristotle*, ed. Richard McKeon (New York: Random House, 1941) (1253a 10–18).

7. See, in particular, the work of R. A. Spitz, "Hospitalism: An Inquiry into the Genesis of Psychiatric Conditions in Early Childhood," *Psychoanalytic Study of the Child* 1 (1945): 53–74, https://doi.org/10.1080/00797308.1945.11823126; and H. F. Harlow, "The Nature of Love," *American Psychologist* 13, no. 12 (1958):673–85, https://doi:10.1037/h0047884.

8. Virginia Held, "Non-contractual Society: A Feminist View," *Canadian Journal of Philosophy*, supp. vol. 13 (1987): 118, 119.

9. Daniel J. Wakin, "Faces That Can't Be Forgotten," *New York Times*, April 16, 2020, https://www.nytimes.com/2020/04/16/reader-center/coronavirus-obits.html.

10. "Missing Them: Remembering the New Yorkers We've Lost to COVID-19," *The City*, https://projects.thecity.nyc/covid-19-deaths/.

PART II

Pandemic, Illness, and Disability

Chapter 4

Sometimes Life Gives You Way Too Many Lemons: An Observation in Nine Parts

Ruth Groenhout

As the COVID-19 pandemic began, I was just about eighteen months past an initial diagnosis of advanced and nasty cancer. But there wasn't just the physical cancer that I had to fight—there was also the political cancer of the Trump presidency with its glorification of racism, bigotry, hatred, and deep injustice. This rose to a deadly level with the protests after the killing of an unarmed, nonviolent black man by four police officers in Minneapolis—a deep cancer in the structure of the nation. Added to this is an emotional and psychological cancer that comes from the dissonance between having been raised in a deeply conservative Christian home to believe that Jesus's words matter and watching conservative Christians completely reject every basic teaching of Jesus Christ. All of this feels past healing at this point. So this chapter reflects on living with cancer, living that way during a time of pandemic and deep social unrest, and the way that a philosopher goes on living, sometimes even goes on hoping, in dark times.

INTRODUCTION

The COVID-19 pandemic has been anxiety inducing for people around the globe. For many of us, this stress and anxiety came on top of a whole range of other worries. In my case, the pandemic arrived on top of a cancer diagnosis that could lead to my death. Thinking about the experience of fighting cancer during the pandemic, and doing this during a time of political tension, led to this paper as a combination of personal autobiographical experience and the philosophical thinking that runs in the background. It has been a time of loss and sadness, but also a time to reflect on the things that are valued and that are worth my time even when facing a whole range of concerns.[1]

The widespread and dangerous flood of the pandemic put many people at serious risk, and I do not consider my own issues worse than many of those others. But the whole situation, for me, did bring back the recognition of the importance of philosophy for my life and for the lives of many people around me. This sounds strange to many people, since philosophy often seems like the least helpful pursuit in a time of conflict. While living through all of this, however, I came to respect philosophical thinking all over again, in part because it does matter, even in difficult times. We need to think carefully about who we are and what we value, and we particularly need to carry out that philosophical thinking when tragedy strikes and we have to face shared challenges.

FIGHTING DEATH DURING A GLOBAL PANDEMIC

> Philosophy isn't something that comes to the soul by accident, for it is nothing other than this vigil over death that watches out for death and watches over death, as if over the very life of the soul.
>
> —Jacques Derrida

I sit in my office at the university with a fabric mask hanging from my neck. Every time I leave the office for any reason, even if it is just to visit the restroom, I tie the mask over my mouth and nose and use hand sanitizer as I leave and as I enter. I try to maintain a certain distance from every other person around. The whole procedure feels excessive, but I am under strict instructions from my doctor to maintain this no matter how it feels. It offers some protection from getting sick, and because of my current health condition, if I get sick, I could easily die. I really don't want to die right now.

The COVID-19 pandemic of 2020 changed the world for everyone. In my particular case, it occurred about eighteen months after a diagnosis of advanced ovarian cancer, the cancer my mother died of and that I inherited as a result of BRCA2 genes. I've gotten through two surgeries, extensive chemotherapy, and then watched the cancer number fly right back up again as soon as I had been off chemo for a few months. So I take what's called a PARP inhibitor, a very new treatment that offers me a chance to live a bit longer. It's not really fun, but it means I could live for five or six more years instead of dying in six months. Frankly, I'm gonna take it.

I am a philosopher by trade and by nature, so all of this becomes something I think about not just in a practical way, but also in terms of the meaning it holds for my sense of self, identity, and questions about what it is to live a good life. Receiving a diagnosis of terminal cancer does push all these questions to the top of my consciousness and makes it extremely difficult to maintain the sort of neutral, distanced discussion of abstract topics that academics prefer. Modern academic structures strongly encourage scholars to stay away from difficult personal questions, although that is a bit less the case in one of my main fields, bioethics. But because I do know a lot about medicine, both its history and practice, and especially know a lot about the ethical issues that are central to the contemporary world of medical matters, dealing firsthand with my medical condition and treatment exists, for me, both at the level of practical decisions as well as of philosophical considerations. The combination of these two can get complicated.

And all of this cancer stuff is occurring within the context of a global pandemic, with the number of COVID cases skyrocketing around the globe, the number of people dying from the disease hitting horrible numbers, and a national response to the problem that is appallingly incompetent. I have worked with committees that considered possible responses to pandemics in the past, and huge portions of the current policies are simply ignoring or even rejecting basic ways of slowing down the spread of the virus and offering adequate treatment to those at risk. This is both a matter of professional nightmares, but also, for me, a very personal fear.

THINKING RATIONALLY IN A CRAZY WORLD

> It requires courage to even leave the protective security of our four walls and enter the public realm, not because of particular dangers which may lie in wait for us, but because we have arrived in a realm where the concern for life has lost its validity. Courage liberates men from their worry about life for the freedom of the world. Courage is indispensable because in politics not life but the world is at stake.
>
> —Hannah Arendt

Because I am taking a medication that diminishes my healing capacity and am also still getting over all the cancer treatment from earlier, if I were to get COVID-19, there is a very good chance it would kill me. My body just doesn't have the healing capacity it would need to fight off the infection. So

I have to make sure I am taking every possible precaution I can while still going to work and coming into contact with all sorts of people, any one of whom could be carrying the virus. There's a level of stress to all this that scares me on a regular basis.

Access to vaccinations has been terribly slow, partly because of how badly (dis)organized the whole pandemic situation has been and partly because of how dangerous the disease is and how many people need to be vaccinated. At the time of this writing, in the particular county of the state in which I currently live, vaccines are being offered to people in "Group One"—people who work in healthcare. They are also offered to "Group Two"—people who are sixty-five or older. No one else is supposed to have access, though rumors are flying about wealthy folks who, while fitting neither of these categories, have gotten the vaccine anyway. The state-level CDC offers a different set of standards for the two groups than my county, particularly Group Two, which it thinks should only be people seventy-five and older, while Group One should include all "frontline workers"—which means everyone in constant contact with lots of people every day.

When I am allowed to get the vaccine, I'll get it by setting up an appointment with my local hospital and then driving through one of the hospital's parking lots, where there are lots of tents and lines set up for drive-throughs. I've driven past that parking lot several times, as it is very close to my home; there are never any cars in it and the tents are frequently not staffed, so one does not get the sense that the vaccine is being provided to lots of people. It is still unclear whether I will fall into "Group Three"—frontline workers, including educators (though some states and some counties are excluding university professors)—or "Group Four"—people at risk from other health conditions, and, well, pretty much everyone else. Why people with already existing health issues are being seated at the very back of this list is unclear, but perhaps we are considered a waste of resources.

SOCIAL STRUCTURES AND PANDEMICS

> [*M*]edical intervention must be understood as an attempt to restore an equilibrium that has been disturbed. It is in this that the genuine "work" of medical art consists.
>
> —Hans-Georg Gadamer

Because I work in bioethics, I know that medical researchers and practitioners have provided extensive planning for dealing with the sort of situation we are confronting and that their planning has simply been thrown away to make a political point. And so I am mourning and angry: mourning the deaths of hundreds of thousands of people, my own citizens, dying from a disease that could have been prevented; angry that those with money and power are approaching a serious emergency without any concern for the people facing death every time they walk into work.

The resistance to the simple acts of wearing masks, handwashing, and social distancing is particularly hard to take and stressful. I happen to live in a county that is heavily populated by people who believe that they should constantly show support for former president Donald Trump by refusing to participate in these basic acts of mutual care. And because so many of my fellow citizens are also lovers of guns and not averse to violence if confronted, store employees, for the most part, simply let them walk in the door without a mask—and I cannot blame them. The employees have to protect themselves from both the virus and the fury of the virus deniers.

Entering Walmart a few weeks ago (Walmart is far worse for this problem than other grocery stores), I found myself behind an older couple, probably in their late sixties or early seventies, both clearly in poor health. Neither wore a mask. Both were coughing as they walked into the store ahead of me, and they made fairly rude comments to the employee who sat at a small table at the entrance, offering free masks to anyone walking in. It's hard to know what feelings such people should elicit. They are clearly endangering themselves—and are proud of it—but they are also endangering lots of other people, and they seem largely unconcerned with that possibility. As I walked right behind them, breathing the air that they were inhaling and exhaling, trying not to touch any of the shopping carts they touched and coughed on, what I did feel was a mixture of compassion and disgust. And while this is probably not particularly virtuous of me, it is honest.

The notion that when life gives one lemons, the right way to approach things is to "make lemonade" has been widespread in popular approaches to anxiety and stress. But a diagnosis of possibly terminal cancer, added to the serious social, economic, and personal costs of a pandemic, is hard to envision as a couple of lemons. Maybe a whole dump truck of lemons descending on me all at once? And if I'm buried in lemons, telling me to make lemonade is not really helpful advice. In fact, it borders on cruel.

The stress is compounded by the other outside contact I experience on a regular basis. I need to continue with work because without a salary it would be extremely hard to pay my medical bills and afford health insurance. It occurs to me quite regularly that I would be much better off living in a country that actually provides realistic access to healthcare for all and doesn't link healthcare to one's employment status. *Sigh.* I was not born into such a country. So I go in to work, I follow the proper procedures, I wear a mask when I grocery shop. I try to behave like the grown up that I am.

What gets hard is not letting the stress of all that get to me. Sleeping at night is difficult. I wake up desperate that I might lose my job, my insurance, and my medicine. If I try to calm my mind about that danger, my brain then jumps to what will happen if I catch the virus, or if my partner or someone else I love catches it.

But, of course, when it rains trouble, there's never just one level of flooding. I live during the time of the (now former) Trump presidency, and the Trump administration's response to the coronavirus has been about as incompetent as anything of the sort could be. Trump refused to listen to his own advisers early on, pretending there was no virus and that nothing needed to be done. And now there is ample evidence that he was informed of the risks and chose to minimize them, to conceal them, to lie about them. He threw out the pandemic planning team the Obama administration left for him and has regularly denied or rejected advice that comes from the national CDC. He constantly denigrated the World Health Organization and finally left it altogether—in the midst of a global pandemic. When the disease numbers started soaring, he advised people to use medicines that offered no help at all, failing completely to provide adequate protective equipment while also insisting that appropriate precautions were being taken. The death toll is now over five hundred thousand and the virus is continuing to spread.

One of the worst moves of the Trump presidency, because it is so visible and contrary to basic evidence, has been the politicization of wearing masks. Partly this has been to appeal to the QAnon enthusiasts who consider the pandemic to be a hoax, partly to appeal to the religious conservatives who are extremely vocal about how their faith removes all fear of disease, and partly in service of his own hubris. Knowing I am at risk, and that people without masks endanger themselves, endanger others, and spread the disease more widely than it needs to be spread, makes all of this rather nauseating. And, unfortunately, that is a literal use of the term nauseating. Stress takes a physical toll, and bearing witness to repeated dangerous actions of others raises stress levels higher still. It's as if there are vises gripping my insides, tightening every time the proud antimaskers strut in their solipsistic denial.

What's worse is that I can't ignore any of this because my focus *is* bioethics. I actually have some knowledge of what a pandemic is and how it works. I've worked hard to get to where I am in my career, and to watch an incompetent president get everything deliberately wrong is horrifying. This is especially so as I teach bioethics in the middle of this disaster to students who want to know the truth. I think I've never in my life come so close to biting off my tongue while trying to sound neutral.

But because this is my area of research, I also know what danger presidential myopia poses to me, to *us*, beyond the coronavirus. The Trump administration's repeated attempts to get the courts to declare the Affordable Care Act unconstitutional continues even as I sit in my office with a mask tied around my neck and hand sanitizer all over my hands. If they are successful, my cancer becomes a preexisting condition, one for which I won't be able to be treated if I ever need to change insurance companies. It will also lead to millions of my fellow citizens losing their insurance automatically in the middle of a pandemic. Many of us are likely to die. Did I already mention that I don't really want to die right now? Seems to be a bit of a theme going on.

All of this is taking place against the backdrop of the ongoing racism that has been a part of the American landscape since its inception. The killing of George Floyd by white police officers who appeared almost bored as they crushed his neck with a knee for almost nine minutes has been followed by massive street protests and increasing police violence, while militia groups, armed and threatening legislators, fail to provoke a similar response. I can't participate in the protests, even if I wear a mask.

While racism and a pandemic do begin as different sorts of social problems, the pandemic spreads when people are in often violent contact with each other and their intersections become intimate and tragic. All sorts of public events—from protests and rallies to sporting events and church services—are implicated, with no safe spaces. How one talks to others in these circumstances gets complicated and stressful.

Issues of racism also make the vaccination process difficult. A significant number of members of the African American community are suspicious of the vaccine for a variety of reasons. It is also the case that the definitions of groups who have access to the vaccine has not been particularly helpful for some portions of the African American community. Who gets defined as a "frontline worker" has sometimes excluded minority groups who are clearly frontline in the sense that they deal with lots of people every day. Again, the situation adds to my concerns and anxiety, but I am not in a position to change things.

FIGHTING FOR JUSTICE IN A TIME OF PANDEMIC

> *The oppressors do not perceive their monopoly on* having more *as a privilege which dehumanizes others and themselves. They cannot see that, in the egoistic pursuit of* having *as a possessing class, they suffocate in their own possessions and no longer* are; *they merely* have. —Paulo Freire

It feels as though the country is fighting cancer collectively at the same time as I fight it individually. By definition, cancer is a condition where the body's own cells become damaging because they refuse to respect the other organs and individual cellular material. Instead, the cancerous cells try to force every cell in the body to support only themselves, just as some people think only their rights and desires count. We see it when they try to take away health insurance (and in the United States, that means healthcare) from millions of citizens while making sure the wealthy pay almost no tax. We see it in removing huge numbers of barriers to pollution being dumped in the groundwater and the air. This happens as wealthy corporations are encouraged to pollute. And we, who depend on the water and air, in turn face horrendous disease and the loss of a general sense of safety. Similarly, the persistent damage and deaths resulting from the pandemic continue to grow with no adequate responses in sight. If these don't sound like a social version of cancer, I'm not sure what does.

This social upheaval, combined with wildly incompetent treatment of a serious global health emergency, serves as a large helping of lemons. Sometimes it feels as though just staying alive, breathing, and functioning at some level from day to day may be more than I can handle. Lemonade just does not seem possible.

THINGS (CAN JUST) FALL APART

> *Folly is a more dangerous enemy to the good than malice. You can protest against malice, you can unmask it or prevent it by force. Malice always contains the seeds of its own destruction, for it always makes men* [*and women*] *uncomfortable, if nothing worse. There is no defense against folly.*
>
> —Dietrich Bonhoeffer

It feels funny, writing all of this. One of the frustrating results of chemotherapy is that it messes with your vocabulary. So as I sit here at my computer, typing away, I regularly have a word or two that I know, have used countless times before, and can't come up with right now. At home, watching birds, I keep calling chickadees "chipmunks." Others seem to find it confusing.

At work, I've learned to just keep writing, putting in a clump of parentheses where the word I'm forgetting can be inserted later. It usually shows up a few minutes later than when I needed it, but I can just fill it in to the blank that I left and keep going. The technique does not work so well when I'm lecturing in a classroom and a word refuses to come to mind. Oh, the joy of teaching after chemotherapy! It is better to suffer occasional awkwardness, however, than to be dead, so if this is the price of survival, I'm still grateful for the chemo.

And the students have really been lovely as I've been working through the diagnosis, treatment, and (sort of) recovery. During the early discovery of the cancer, after I returned with the initial diagnosis, several students stopped by as they were leaving the classroom and told me they were praying for me. It was so well meant and so generous, and I thought they were sweet. They were even nice enough to ask if it was okay if they prayed for me, which struck me as pretty high-level recognition, and acceptance, of differences.

But while those prayers felt like positive generosity and were valued, they also came into a world where prayer has become something else altogether. Trump's most vocal supporters these days come from white Evangelical churches. This is a world I know a lot about, because I was raised a missionary kid and spent summers being hauled around from one church to another by my parents. In all those white Evangelical churches that we visited, and in so many yet today, prayer is always the response to any worries, disasters, or problems. My mom, being a missionary for so much of her life, got prayers beyond belief when she was diagnosed with ovarian cancer. She died within six months of the diagnosis, and so far as anyone can tell, the prayers did absolutely nothing. Her death was lonely, painful, and awful.

But this is where things get murkier in the white Evangelical church. First, there's the classic philosophical problem of evil. Both my mom and I have a cancer that is caused by a genetic condition—BRCA2—which makes prayers extraordinarily problematic. Think about it for a second: The source of our cancer isn't something that can be blamed on evil choices that humans have made; instead, the source of the cancer has been created by whoever or whatever created all of reality. That's how genetic material works. So if the God that Christian theology preaches exists, that's who is the creator of, and the reason for, our cancer. After all, it is basic Christian theology that God is the creator of all that exists, and nothing exists that God did not create. Traditionally, this generates what philosophers call "the problem of evil"—questions such as: Where does evil come from if a good God is the source of all existence? Why would an absolutely good and all-powerful being create evil things? One of the most important Christian theologians/philosophers, St. Augustine, argued that the proper understanding is that evil is not something that exists. It is, by definition, a lack of existence—a loss of the proper structures in reality that generates really bad results.

I know good old Augustine well and have taught the problem of evil to students for years. But the situation here—a cancer that is caused by a genetic condition—is exactly the sort of case that causes deep problems for this account of the nature of evil. After all, if the cancerous genetic condition is created by God, and if Augustine is right, then we have two options. Either (1) this cancer is actually a good thing (Hey, God created it!) or (2) it is a bad thing (It is a nasty, painful and horrible way to die, there are no cures, and one gets it late in life after it has been passed on to the next generation). If we start with option 1, then we are stuck with a God who deliberately chose to create a really nasty condition because to that God, that condition is a good thing. Sadism—watching people die painful and unnecessary deaths that one has willingly created—doesn't fit well with the claim that God is good. But if we go the other way, we are stuck with either the notion that lots of stuff exists that God did not create (which allows God to be good, but not the creator of all, so it doesn't fit with Christian theology) or that we are somehow supposed to mesh the idea that God is good with the idea that God deliberately chose to create horrible stuff—and we are back to option 1.

HOW TO THINK ABOUT EVIL?

> In an age in which the ancient sense of solidarity was crumbling and the individual experienced his sufferings in that utter solitude which is now once again the mark of modernity, the author of Job refused all the comforts that go with the assurance that God is perfectly merciful and just—the promises that being moral pays either in this life or the next—and, with a radicalism that has parallels in Amos and the other prophets of his type, but scarcely in the Gospels, claimed that God was neither just nor the embodiment of mercy or perfection.
>
> —Walter Kaufmann

This does, of course, represent one of the difficulties of being a philosopher dealing with cancer, whether cancer of the body, of the social world, or of the soul. The bodily cancer is just not something we can make fit with standard theological claims about God, and philosophers tend to be just really, really bad about ignoring those contradictions and continuing to believe no matter what. But the social cancers are no different. We know that the Holocaust generated deep loss of faith in so many because if a good, all-powerful God actually existed, why would that God fail to intervene? And when the Holocaust was followed by Stalinist purges in the Soviet Union, Jim Crow laws and continued lynching of African Americans in the United States, and then horrific ethnic cleansing in far too many countries around the globe, the horror gets worse and worse.

In the contemporary world, there's a particularly nasty version of this problem that is generated by white Evangelical support of Trump. When someone claiming to be a follower of Jesus Christ publicly claims that *nothing* will cause them to cease their support for a man who is anything but Christlike, that person has moved into what standard Christian theology considers idolatry. They have made a false God and have allowed him to define reality, such as the claims that drinking bleach would help cure coronavirus or that packed political rallies are harmless, simply because he said so. And so I wonder: What does it take for an individual to see past the lies, past the propaganda? And as the people who got sick at these rallies then pass on the coronavirus to vulnerable family members, very little recognition by the adoring throngs was in evidence.

CONTRADICTIONS AND HEALTHY THINKING

> *Whence is it that [fools] are in so great request with Princes . . . ? [F]ools fit 'em with what they most delight in, as jests, laughter, abuses of other men, wanton pastimes, and the like.*
>
> —Desiderius Erasmus

Now consider that white Evangelicals make up a huge percentage of those who allow Trump to define reality and morality. These are individuals who claim to be believers in the Christian God, who claim to be followers of Jesus Christ, while literally selling their souls to an individual who seems to care only about his own power. Again, being a philosopher makes this enormously uncomfortable, because deep contradictions are very hard for philosophers to ignore. One can worship Trump and claim that freedom of religion allows this. That's certainly true. One can worship Jesus Christ, again based on freedom of religion and a commitment to the basic teachings of Jesus found in the gospels of Matthew, Mark, Luke, and John. What one cannot do is claim that doing both of these at the same time is possible. Jesus taught that one should love and care for the poor, the sick, the vulnerable; Trump doesn't care if the sick die and the poor are both starving and faced with extremely high risk of COVID-19. Jesus taught a God of truth; Trump's constant lying promotes bigotry and hatred of people who bear God's image. One can choose to worship either of these gods, but not both.

So when I'm offered prayers from white Evangelicals, and especially when prayer, in their mind, is the only thing one ever offers those needing help, it rings pretty hollow. But one of the effects of all of this is that I have lost any and all religious faith during this time—and, again, as a philosopher, I am unable to simply ignore what looks pretty obviously true in order to just go on believing something false.

This deep loss of faith is coming at a particularly hard time for me. Dealing with possibly terminal cancer during the time of a highly politicized global pandemic is a ton of lemons to have dumped on me all at once. Doing this while also losing any ability to trust that there is a good and loving God, or that there is deep meaning in human life, takes away one of the support networks that humans have often turned to. The loss is real and deep, generating both despair and mourning. I spent so much of my life serving the needs of the faith and of the church, and to have all that made worthless at this point in my life is another huge truckload of lemons.

Unfortunately, dear reader, I also have just dumped a ton of negativity on you.

And it points to the problem: One cannot make lemonade when one feels like one has become an exhausted, empty jug. Even more relevant, the story of "making lemonade" is a narrative of toxic optimism. It demands that people dealing with exhausting stress and fear should "lighten the load" for everyone else, and so it adds insult to injury. One of the things that has made it so hard for the United States to produce a coherent pandemic plan is precisely the tendency for the country to insist that individuals always need to solve their own problems rather than looking for collective responses: Changing the social structures in the United States has real value; standing up against racist police violence has real value. But I am not an optimist.

GLIMMERS OF HOPE ON THE HORIZON

> *The continued pursuit of a major intellectual process by* [*humans*] *requires a state of social dedication and . . . only in a dedicated society can* [*humans*] *live an intellectually and morally acceptable life. This cannot fail to suggest that the whole purpose of society lies in enabling its members to pursue their transcendent obligations; particularly to truth, justice, and charity.*
>
> —Michael Polanyi

Any reference to hope at this point may sound naive. I've just been going on and on about the pain in so much of our shared and unshared experiences, calling them cancer. But one of the important things to remember about cancer is that a healthy body can actually fight back against certain types of cancer cells. My own cancer is one that can be partially tracked by taking blood and counting the number of CA125 cells present from one time to the next. And even healthy people have a low number of these CA125 cells all the time. My numbers went down to that healthier range while I was going through chemo, only to jump back up after only a few months because my cancer is quite resistant to chemo. Yet many healthy people are walking around with low levels of cancer cells in their body, able to live normal lives, never having to deal with tumors growing—never actually having a case of ovarian cancer.

The reason for this is that other cells in the body treat the cancer cells as something to keep under control, not something to allow to grow and take over. That to me is an analogy that fits the social world, too. There will always be people who really don't care in the slightest about fairness, equality, or decent protection of the vulnerable. But a healthy society keeps those voices to a fairly limited range. Unfortunately, the current world has moved to a situation where the harmful values have taken on enormous power. Those who have made QAnon their source of information and sold themselves to social movements based on lies, a sense of victimization, rejection of basic moral values, and racism need to be recognized as poisonous to society. The rest of the population needs to protect themselves from these types and speak loudly about the importance of actual facts, understanding how reason works, being committed to protecting basic rights for all people, and respecting the rule of law. Instead, we have a group that (as I am writing this chapter) created a mob and broke into the halls of Congress with the intent of harming congressional members doing their constitutional duty. This is something that needs to be kept from growing.

The arrival of COVID-19 to the country has forced a reckoning with the cost of destroying basic principles of justice and fairness. Employees who we really cannot live without (grocery store workers, meat plant workers, healthcare workers) are declared "essential" while working for ridiculously low pay at jobs that put them in serious danger of contracting the virus. If they are essential, why do we not pay them decent wages? Why are the rich owners of the corporations that hire them, rich people who do very little to keep the world running, allowed to force them to sign waivers that prevent them from suing if they get coronavirus while working under unsafe conditions? Basic conceptions of fairness and protection of basic rights—these are issues that come up time after time during the pandemic.

Yet ethics has not left me in the way that religion has. It is not perfect—nothing we humans do is perfect—but over the centuries, there have been individuals who cared enough about the difference between right and wrong, between the values that should structure human life and those that should not, to allow us to ask hard questions about why we live the way we do and whether there are other ways of doing that would be better. It's almost as if the philosophers are part of this white blood cell contingent of society at large, asking the questions that need to be asked. And when the philosophers, in turn, are effective, they don't insist that the only answer to social problems is to pursue perfection. Instead, they recognize that we need systems that are better than the alternatives and that generally work reasonably well. They know that lemons sometimes have to be seen for what they are.

WHAT PHILOSOPHY OFFERS

> [*Absolute purity*] is one bad but common approach to devastation in all its forms. It is a common approach for anyone who attempts to meet and control a complex situation that is fundamentally outside our control. It is a bad approach because it shuts down precisely the field of possibility that might allow us to take better collective action against the destruction of the world in all its strange, delightful, impure frolic.
>
> —Alexis Shotwell

Thinking that the only good way to live under all these conditions is to pursue absolute perfection, or to assume that this should be our goal, is just wrong. Confused and myopic citizens will probably always be with us, and they deserve basic human rights just like everyone else. Trying to force them to care about truth is likely to backfire horrendously. Likewise, recognizing that the cancer I now face requires me to take medicine that is really not good for the rest of my cells doesn't make the medicine bad, evil, or the vicious development of Big Pharma—it makes the complicated reality of life something that cannot be ignored.

So working through the philosophical solutions allows me to get some distance from the raucous noise of the scary world we live in and to think about the wide-ranging ways that human communities have developed to be relatively healthy, even in difficult times. We live at a time in history when we can actually learn from our past, and there are clearly some answers that work better than others. One of the obvious ones is supporting people who keep society running while limiting the spread of cancerous beliefs and actions.

And philosophy offers a second reason to hope: the younger generation, refusing to buy into ignorance, racism, and hatred. One of the reasons for this refusal is the change that university education can provide. When students read a wide range of books and research articles; when they find themselves sitting next to people from all sorts of class, race, and ethnic groups; when they discover that others' definitions of gender and sexuality may not be what they grew up with, they can shift into a diversity-embracing worldview that does not require people to defend their own identity solely through the hatred of others.

Part of what a body needs to fight cancer is also a diverse range of different cells, each of them becoming a particular kind of thing that is not the same as the other cells around it. Liver cells are quite different from bone cells. White blood cells do not look or function like gall bladder cells. Even though they all come from the same source—all have the same DNA and all could be traced back to the original embryo from which they developed—they've all gone in different directions of development and identity. And it is precisely *because* they are all different that the body works. Cancer tries to force them all into becoming one type of thing. That is why it kills.

Socially, there's a lot to recognize here. People do all share human nature, but society isn't healthy when all humans are forced to fit into one simplistic set of categories. A community needs a whole range of people, each becoming what they should be, not forced into exactly the same mold in every case. On top of this, recognizing how many different ways there are to live, seeing the fun in doing life in wildly different ways and celebrating the range of human identity, is essential to learning what it can mean to be human.

HOW THINKING HELPS US KEEP GOING

> If it happens that, here or there, we are capable of thinking that peace is possible where conflict mesmerizes us, and reduces us to impotence, "think we must."
>
> —Isabelle Stengers and Vinciane Despret

This week has been a particularly stressful one. All the levels of cancer are active. On the personal level, I needed to go into the hospital for blood work and a CT scan to see if, or how much, the cancer is progressing. Nothing like getting needles inserted into your body to really feel good! Even entering the health context requires wearing a mask, getting temperatures taken outside, answering all sorts of odd questions. This week's responses included: "No, I have not been in or visited a prison or jail in the last two weeks." Good Lord! So the weirdness of the cultural level of the horrific spread of the coronavirus spreads also from the more political dimension into my personal life.

Yet there are still points of light that break in, and they come from such a surprising place: from my work in philosophy, remembering philosophers who feed my soul, reading new ones who offer a way to keep moving forward in all of this, even when it looks as though the cancer has spread to far too many places.

Early on in my education, I was introduced to a relatively minor philosopher, Epictetus, whose basic Stoic approach held meaning then and still helps me today. How a man writing philosophy that was designed to help his fellow citizens make their lives good human lives in the era of the Roman empire could have said something that still resonates today, I don't know. But he was, among other things, honest and straightforward. You don't control your world, I don't control mine, he wrote, because we live in a world that started before we existed and will exist after we are gone. But the first step in having a life worth living is to recognize and accept that the vast majority of what occurs, in my body, in my society, in my religious communities, is completely independent of anything I can do or think. It is not up to me.

Yet there are things that are up to me. I am the one who chooses what to connect my emotions to, what values are going to matter to me. That choice is absolutely mine, one for which I am the most responsible. And if that is my choice, I'd better make it well. For Epictetus, making that choice well required removing any emotional connections to things that are completely outside my control. If those things control my emotions, then I know, without any logical uncertainty, that my emotions are going to be of the negative variety because the world isn't going to somehow conform to what I want. It's time to grow up and acknowledge this. But I can connect my emotions to things that I do have some control over, and I can discipline those emotions so that they respond to those things as they are. Sometimes this is easy. Epictetus offers the example of a little pottery jug that I look at and enjoy using, but whose breakability I also must accept. When it breaks, I will say, "That's what jugs do," and feel no sorrow or loss because I knew all along how jugs work.

But Epictetus also thinks exactly the same response should occur when things are hard. When I look at my son, he thought, I should accept that while I love him now, I also need to see clearly that he is a mortal human being and will die one day. And when he dies, I should say, "That's what mortals do," and feel no sorrow or loss.

Now here is where I part ways with old Epictetus, because I think he misses one more step in accepting the realities of the world we live in. I love my son, and when I think about his possible death, I also need to see that physical, mortal, biological beings like me and my son have deep and important emotional connections that generate deep sorrow when there is loss. This isn't just some random choice; it's the very nature of biological social beings, and that means that I need to see clearly our relationship as full of both joy and sadness—and that this is how it should be. So while I've never bought Epictetus's idea that the death of a child shouldn't be mourned, I do think an honest recognition of human life accepts the sorrows involved in losses of what, and who, matters.

All disagreements aside, Epictetus offers an important way of moving forward during times when no control is possible. I can take all the medicine my doctor gives me, but I know that death is coming way earlier than I wanted it and that I can stave it off only for so long. I can vote, support protesters, do everything I can to support sensible approaches to the pandemic, but I am only one fairly small person in a huge country filled with other people, many of whom hold the kinds of views that I find not only abhorrent, but existentially threatening. I can't change that. I can write essays that clearly argue that positions held and funded by white Evangelical Trump worshippers are clearly anti-Christian views. But they won't read the essays, and even if they did, they would dismiss my words. And I have no control over that.

What I do control, however, is whether I allow the events happening around me to consume me emotionally. I can let my soul be destroyed, or I can set that aside, denying them their power. This choice is mine. And, again, it puts our lemonade in context. I can't turn the hard and violent events occurring in my country into happy thoughts. Lemonade is not the right approach. But I can recognize what I am able to respond to and what I cannot respond to, and I can recognize how many people are fighting the cancer in our world and be really grateful for them. Accepting my own finitude and accepting that I am not responsible for how this whole story plays out is an important part of maintaining sanity through these days and months of pandemic. And I have philosophy, in part, to thank for this.

CONCLUSION(?)

As I am finishing this chapter, Congress is holding the second impeachment trial for the former president, showing videos of the mob breaking into the halls of Congress, beating the police officers trying to hold them at bay, and searching for senators and representatives who could be attacked. And the Trump supporters in the very Congress that was attacked are preparing to simply ignore it all. The social cancer runs deep.

Yet when life presents us with horrors, the right response is to recognize that they are horrible. We need to accept that mourning and sorrow and anxiety are appropriate responses to some of what occurs in the world. And so my friends who have lost loved family members to the pandemic need to mourn those losses, full stop. We need to care about truth and reason and respond with the appropriate emotions. A part of that truth is that evil does actually occur, and unless we recognize and address it *as such*, we become complicit.

The sky outside my window this afternoon is dark grey, foggy and drizzly. Perhaps the right response is not to rail against the lack of sunlight but to let ourselves mourn, to support and care for those who are suffering and who need help, and to try to understand the difference between what can, and what cannot, be changed. Forget trying to make lemonade. Respond honestly, kindly, responsibly. Let yourself cry. Let others cry. And then resolve to build the kind of world that moves us all toward greater health, deeper solidarity, and broader compassion.

CITATIONS

Jacques Derrida, *The Gift of Death*, trans. David Wills (Chicago: University of Chicago Press, 1995), 15.

Hannah Arendt, *Between Past and Future: Eight Exercises in Political Thought* (New York: Penguin Books, 1954; 1977), 156.

Hans-Georg Gadamer, *The Enigma of Health: The Art of Healing in a Scientific Age*, trans. Jason Gaiger and Nicholas Walker (Stanford, CA: Stanford University Press, 1996), 36.

Paulo Freire, *Pedagogy of the Oppressed*, trans. Myra Bergman Ramos (New York: Continuum Press, 1970; 1992), 45.

Dietrich Bonhoeffer, *Letters and Paper from Prison*, ed. Eberhard Bethge, trans. Reginald Fuller (New York: MacMillan, 1953; 1965), 22.

Walter Kaufmann, *The Faith of a Heretic* (New York: Doubleday Anchor 1961; 1963), 155–56.

Desiderius Erasmus, *The Praise of Folly*, with a short life of the author by Hendrick Willem van Loon of Rotterdam (New York: Walter J. Black, 1942), 152.

Alexis Shotwell, *Against Purity: Living Ethically in Compromised Times* (Minneapolis: University of Minneapolis Press, 2016) pp. 8–9.

Isabelle Stengers, Vinciane Despret, and collective, *Women Who Make a Fuss: The Unfaithful Daughters of Virginia Woolf*, trans. April Knutson (Minneapolis; Univocal, 2014), 66.

Michael Polanyi, *Science, Faith, and Society* (Chicago: University of Chicago Press, 1946; 1964), 83.

NOTE

1. My thanks to Anna Gotlib for all the work of editing that has gone into this project, and into this paper. Many of the positive aspects of this chapter are due to Gotlib, while any negatives are due to me.

Chapter 5

The Nightmare of Triage and Discrimination: Whose Benefit Is to be Maximized?

Eva Feder Kittay[1]

In April 2020 I wrote:

> I have nightmares, whether asleep or awake—as do we all as we endure the trials of the pandemic. Will it strike us, our families or friends? Who will get sick, very sick, or die? Will we or our loved ones be alone as the disease does its worst, and will we or those we care about be left to die alone? It's less the social isolation that weighs on us as the fear of being isolated from those we love—in illness and in death.[2]

In June 2020, we would read stories that realized this nightmare. This one comes from Washington state:

> At Christmastime last December, Sharon Gowdey was a healthy 56-year-old woman with Down syndrome. A video from a holiday party shows her in a Santa hat dancing to a Michael Jackson song as strobe lights light up the dance floor. . . . Four months later, Gowdey was dead of COVID-19.
>
> "When they turned the ventilator off, it was less than five minutes and she passed away," said her sister Kathleen Hesseltine. . . . Hesseltine recalled that one day they were having lunch in Gowdey's back yard at a safe distance. A couple of days later her sister was calling her. "And she didn't sound right," Hesseltine said. Gowdey soon tested positive for COVID-19 and was hospitalized. Since Hesseltine wasn't allowed to visit, she and her sister communicated by FaceTime. Initially, it seemed like Gowdey would make it through. But a

few days into her hospital stay, the situation turned dire. Hesseltine said it was unbelievable how quickly the virus took over.[3]

It is now one year since I wrote the "The First Opinion" for *STAT*. One year ago, the uncertainty, the timeline, the possible havoc the virus could wreak had brought to mind the tsunami of December 26, 2004, that followed a 9.1-magnitude quake off the northern tip of Sumatra in Indonesia. It washed away bartender, waitress, cleaning staff, and happy tourists who were enjoying a day at a spectacular beach resort in Bali. It was a searing picture: scores of vacationers and residents standing at the edge of a beach, watching in amazement as the water rushed back into the ocean before it returned with a force that swept them and thousands upon thousands away with its stunning force.

In April 2020, it felt as if we were sitting on that sand beach watching and waiting for tsunami. Today we have seen the devastation the pandemic has and is still causing—our world remains topsy-turvy even as some of us are starting to remember what life was like before.

Today, my daughter returns home on weekends, as she has done nearly every weekend since she moved into her group home. This comes after nearly a full year of glimpsing her mostly on FaceTime. The agency that runs her home has not suffered any fatalities and has seen only a very few mild cases. They have vaccinated all residents under their care, and most of their staff. This has been achieved in the face of horrible statistics regarding people with intellectual and developmental disabilities, especially in congregate settings. This population is six times as likely to get ill and twice as likely to die. Their success has come with a high price, both monetarily and emotionally. The distance and isolation have been very difficult for all involved. But my daughter and the rest of the people in her community are alive and extremely unlikely to now need hospitalization and risk death—the stuff of my nightmares.

Many strictures remain despite the high vaccination rate. The many families who cannot bring their child or sibling home can have only very short scheduled visits.

And even though our daughter is vaccinated, we still have to deal with the looming fear of hospitalization from other causes given the continuation of the pandemic. As medical personnel are stretched thin and exhausted—and as some lifesaving resources are in short supply—the prospect of a hospital stay for medically fragile people such as my daughter is still chilling.

Many disabled people and families of those with significant mental or cognitive disability continue to live with the nightmare. For such vulnerable people who are not vaccinated, the fear that the outcome of the illness and hospitalization will almost certainly be tragic continues.[4] The anxiety is not unwarranted. Compounding this vulnerability is the threat that triage protocols will further disadvantage this population. Some of the worst protocols have been modified, but they are still worth considering, since the attitudes that shaped them have not altered.

For example, the original state triage protocols of Alabama explicitly stated that intellectual or cognitive disabilities disqualify a person from treatment when scarce medical resources need to be rationed. ProPublica reports:

> Alabama's plan says that "persons with severe mental retardation, advanced dementia or severe traumatic brain injury may be poor candidates for ventilator support." Another part says that "persons with severe or profound mental retardation, moderate to severe dementia, or catastrophic neurological complications such as persistent vegetative state are unlikely candidates for ventilator support."[5]

Three other states—Kansas, Tennessee, and Washington—had policies sufficiently worrying for disability advocates to file formal complaints with the federal government. And at least twenty other states allow for questionable practices. In one such case, disability advocates have claimed that New York State's 2015 policy on ventilators has permitted hospitals to take them away from disabled patients who must use them in daily life if there is a shortage of ventilators for use in COVID patients.[6]

The federal administration, in response to some state protocols for rationing healthcare during the COVID-19 pandemic, released a statement declaring that no one should be denied treatment because of a disability.[7] We already know that discrimination against people with disabilities violates the law as set down by the Americans with Disabilities Act (ADA) of 1990[8] and the Affordable Care Act (ACA; also known as Obamacare).

My daughter, had she gotten ill and been treated under Alabama-like exclusions, would have no hope. Her cognitive disability is such that her physicians said she has "no measurable IQ." I take this to mean that there are no means of testing her IQ, but strangers would take this to mean that there is no intelligence there to be tested. Yet she lights up my life and those around who get to know her. Her calm, steady loveliness makes the world itself a more beautiful place. She loves her life, which is filled with music, love, and joy. The fact that she cannot speak, cannot walk unassisted, cannot dress or feed or toilet herself, does not give her any less of a right to be in this world, to be respected, to be accorded dignity and given the same level of care as another—even in a pandemic such as the one we face.

When we are dealing with a pandemic where transmissibility rates are as high as they are for COVID-19, the cruelty of the disease is compounded when family members cannot be with their loved ones. Perhaps the worst nightmare of all is that I will not be permitted to be with my daughter if she becomes ill. Will I be barred because we need to save as many lives as possible? Without me, she is unlikely to live. Whose benefits matter? Which lives matter?

Fortunately, many hospitals have recognized that for people with disabilities, especially those who have difficulties in communication, having a family member or caregiver present is essential. I would argue that it is at least as essential as a ventilator is for a vent user. Especially when it comes to interfacing with a professional world, we are the relevant prosthesis—we are the voice, the translator, and the protector that stands in place of her own inability to self-preserve.

Despite the protections of the ADA and antidiscriminatory provisions of the ACA, as well as directives that came from the White House, the fear of triage protocols remains, not only for people with intellectual and developmental disabilities but also for disabled people more generally. Hospitalization, especially in the midst of crisis, even without triage protocols, is a frightening prospect.

People such as my daughter, and many with intellectual disabilities, especially those that are the result of a genetic anomaly, often have medical fragilities (as do many disabled people who have no cognitive impairments). Most doctors and nurses know little about the complexities of a person such as my daughter. And in the context of a pandemic, where they are overwhelmed, understaffed, and exhausted, one cannot expect that they will take the time to understand how to care for her. For example, there are critical knowledge gaps regarding how COVID-19 interacts with her epilepsy or whether medications they supply interact with any of her multiple seizure medications. The staff might not even realize that she cannot follow instructions to "turn over," "take a deep breath," or a number of other standard commands. Will they attempt to treat her at all? If she had a tracheotomy and used a ventilator, will they deploy it for another patient? And perhaps worst of all, will they insist that isolation protocols require that I cannot be there as her advocate, her translator, and her support? A person such as my daughter cannot survive a hospital stay, especially given the nature of *this* disease, without someone who can serve these roles. And this, in fact, may be the case with many others who do not fit the standard model of a patient.

Rationing and triage protocols aggravate an already stomach-churning fear. For even in the absence of overt discrimination, we have to be concerned about the many ways discrimination is baked into standard practices and protocols. Disability activists and organizations have already identified some of the poison pills in seemingly rational recommendations, especially the recommendation to save as many lives as is possible.

Take one example: A standard recommendation is that people with "coexisting health conditions" should have a low priority or should not be treated at all. While a disability itself cannot be considered a coexisting condition, discrimination creeps into the practice of limiting treatment to people even without coexisting conditions, such as lung or heart disease. For instance, many genetic syndromes that cause intellectual, cognitive, or communication disorders also cause scoliosis (that is, curvature of the spine). If the curvature is sufficiently pronounced, it can affect the function of internal organs, especially the lungs, making these individuals more prone to pneumonia, even in the absence of lung disease per se. Similarly, consider the epilepsy that can accompany mental disabilities. Seizures are often triggered by fever. Will this count as a coexisting condition since seizures will make any significant medical treatment more challenging? Furthermore, many intellectually disabled people are unable to follow standard medical directions such as "take a deep breath." Is that not an obstacle to a good prognosis?

Fundamentally, triage protocols are enacted to maximize benefits, following standard utilitarian logic that we need to provide the greatest good for the greatest number. This stands in contrast to the medical standard to provide the best possible care for the patient in the physician's care. In conditions of crisis, there is a strong pull away from the traditional medical standard to utilitarian calculations.

Utilitarian triage protocols function differently when the baseline of the people whose interests are being weighed is very similar and the only significant difference between the individuals is their chance of survival. The soldiers wounded in battle, for example, prior to the injuries sustained in war, are similar in age, ability, and health. A benefit for one soldier is more or less the same as a benefit for another soldier. A calculus determining the greatest good for the greatest number may be the only fair way of allocating the medical care available. There is also a lesser chance that morally irrelevant difference will play a part, although in an army that is racially, sexually, and religiously diverse, there may be danger of bias.

But medical crises such as the pandemic affect a very diverse population. Here, it is clear that benefits are not free-floating goods to be readily counted and divided. Benefits attach to someone.

What this suggests is that a benefit for one may not be a benefit for another. Given baseline differences in age, previous health status, social capital, and ability/disability, the definition of what a "benefit" is becomes rather fluid and context dependent. Is saving a young, unencumbered person a greater benefit (and benefit to whom?) than saving an older person with multiple responsibilities to others? Are the years of life after sixty-five of less value than the same number of years for a forty-year-old? And who is to determine the benefit of cure for someone who is otherwise disabled or has a terminal illness? So we need to ask: "*Whose* 'benefits'? *Who* determines what a benefit looks like? What sort of *calculus* can determine when benefits are maximized? And *who* makes that determination?"

One can reply that the benefit sought in the case of scarce resources is to save as *many* people as possible, something that is countable. Yet in speaking of ventilator allocation, an article in the *Journal of Medical Ethics* points out that translating this "intuitively appealing" principle into "a policy that allocates ventilators to patients who are expected to make faster recoveries puts those who have pre-existing health conditions at a disadvantage. Poor health is affected by, inter alia, age, disability, socio-economic status and genetic luck which may not themselves be fair grounds for rationing"[9].

Indeed, this calculus is unlikely to benefit disabled people. It surely will not benefit people with intellectual disabilities. How many disabled lives will be cut short by protocols that do not consider the impact of recommendations on disabled people? If disabled people—or, in the case of people such as my daughter who cannot speak for themselves, parents or other advocates—do not have a seat at the table, the utilitarian poison pills will go unnoticed or unremarked upon. But the disabled and their families are generally not the authors, the ones who are "in the room where it happens." They determine neither whose benefits are served, nor what the benefits are, nor who does the calculations and how they are made.

Why do the benefits of disabled people seem to count for so little? Why are positive steps taken to protect disabled people, including those with mental disabilities, not considered beneficial in themselves as a part of the overall calculus? The most indecent of societies, Nazi Germany, began its attempt to "purify the race" and rid the world of non-Aryans by killing off mentally disabled people—they then went on to eliminate those lives that *they* decided were unworthy. And as appalling a shocking as we find their crimes, why do we then not count the decency of our own society as a benefit to be added into the calculus—as something to be protected, encouraged, and made central to our reasoning and our actions?

It is worth noting that the talk of allocating preventive vaccines has differed from that which dominates the scarce lifesaving resources for people who have already been infected. I mentioned that my daughter and all the residents covered by her agency have been vaccinated. In fact, they were among the earliest of those vaccinated. The nursing homes with the same residents who would be put last in many protocols received the vaccine before the otherwise healthy forty-year-old who contracted COVID-19. The biblical phrase kept running through my mind: "He who comes last shall come first and he who comes first will be last."

But vaccines, just like ventilators and beds in intensive care units, are equally scarce medical resources. Why the inversion? I believe it is because when we speak of triage, we are speaking of who will survive and return to "normal." When we are considering vaccine allocation, the discussion turns to vulnerability—not who is most likely to live if the medical intervention occurs, but who is most likely to die without the critical vaccines. The baseline medical consideration about who gets treatment if ill is normalcy (normal health, normal capacities, normal functioning). The disabled person, especially those with cognitive disabilities, will not go "back" to normal since that normal never applied to them in the first place. Conversely, the baseline for eligibility for the vaccine is the vulnerability to disease and death. In the case of vaccines, we are not trying to get someone back to normal functioning—we are looking to simply keep those most in danger from dying. These are, if you will, two very different sides of medicine.

Nonetheless, while it was widely recognized that those in Black and Brown communities (as well as prisons and detentions centers) were getting sicker and dying at higher rates than whites and those in wealthier ZIP codes, vaccines did *not* go first to these most vulnerable populations. Also, while some states prioritized those in nursing homes and long-term care facilities, others did not. Not all who came last now came first. It is worth pondering why this divergence occurred. I think the answer might be that there were two sorts of considerations in vaccine distribution: The first was vulnerability, but the second was the degree of importance those in power attached to the lives that would be saved. When the calculus operated only with the first variable, those most vulnerable came first. When the second variable was operative, we got a different outcome. The failure to equally value certain lives, which could so easily taint triage protocols based on returning someone to full functioning, has needed to operate more covertly in the case of vaccines.

Even as there has been much hand-wringing about the difficulty of getting the vaccines into Black and Brown communities and into scarcely populated rural communities, there has been scarcely any about the high death rate and need for vaccines for disabled, especially cognitively disabled. On a rhetorical level at least, we know that "Black Lives Matter." I think we lack even the rhetorical commitment to "Disabled Lives Matter." Thus, we return to some of the questions raised by triage protocols that put disabled people at the end of the queue.

When we ask who arrogates to themselves the determination of what counts as a benefit, we too often and too easily encounter arrogance on the part of those who judge the value of disabled lives. Most able people—and it is generally this group that determines what a benefit looks like—will view a disabled life as a sad, even tragic fate, and with that view, they are likely to discount the benefit and meaning that life produces. Yet studies have consistently shown that *from the disabled person's perspective*, those with very significant disabilities, even intellectual disabilities, can and do live lives of fulfillment, love, and meaning. How good that life is depends on many factors, not least of which is the public perception of the value of that life. The thought that a skewed public perception makes its way into protocols of how medical care is allocated under crisis conditions is, for disabled people and those who care about them, the stuff of nightmares.

NOTES

1. A shorter version of this chapter originally appeared online in *STAT* (https://www.statnews.com) in April 2020 and was reprinted in *Hospital News* (https://hospitalnews.com) and Quoi Media (https://quoimedia.com).

2. Eva Feder Kittay, "People with Disabilities Are at a Disadvantage when Scarce Medical Resources Are Being Allocated," *STAT*, April 29, 2020, https://www.statnews.com/2020/04/29/people-disabilities-disadvantage-covid-19-scarce-medical-resources/.

3. Austin Jekins, "Why Is COVID-19's Death Toll So High for People With Developmental Disabilities?" Oregon Public Broadcasting, June 23, 2020.

4. M. A. Turk, S. D. Landes, M. K. Formica, and K. D. Goss, "Intellectual and Developmental Disability and COVID-19 Case-Fatality Trends: TriNetX Analysis," *Disability and Health Journal* 13, no. 3 (2020): 100942, https://doi.org/10.1016/j.dhjo.2020.100942; S. D. Landes, M. A. Turk, M. K. Formica, K. E. McDonald, and J. D. Stevens, "COVID-19 Outcomes among People with Intellectual and Developmental Disability Living in Residential Group Homes in New York State," *Disability and Health Journal* 13, no. 4 (2020): 100969, https://doi.org/10.1016/j.dhjo.2020.100969; Dalton Stevens and Scott D. Landes, "Potential Impacts of COVID-19 on Individuals with Intellectual and Developmental Disability: A Call for Accurate Cause of Death Reporting," *Research Brief* (Lerner Center for Publica Health Promotion) no. 20 (April 14, 2020).

5. Amy Silverman, "People eith Intellectual Disabilities May Be Denied Lifesaving Care under These Plans as Coronavirus Spreads," Arizona Daily Star, March 27, 2020.

6. New York State Department of Health, New York State Task Force on Life and the Law, "Ventilator Allocation Guidelines," November 2015, https://www.documentcloud.org/documents/6824983-New-York-Ventilator-Guidelines. The problem arises when chronically ill individuals who are users of vents need acute hospital care because they are ill with the virus. If they are triaged in the same manner as non-ventilator users, the criteria may determine that they should not be given a ventilator and so be subject to having their ventilator taken away. They may be denied the use of their ventilator, which would be used by someone who has higher priority in the triage protocol. However, this would likely result in their death, irrespective of their COVID-19 infection. Joseph Fins, a member of the task force, refuted this characterization of the recommendations. In a discussion about reallocation, the authors point to the exchange between disability advocates and Fins as an example of the need

for clarity and transparency. Also see Joel Michael Reynolds, Laura Guidry-Grimes, and Katie Savin, "Against Personal Ventilator Reallocation," *Cambridge Quarterly of Healthcare Ethics* 30, no. 2 (April 2021). Reynolds, J., Guidry-Grimes, L., & Savin, K. (2021). "Against Personal Ventilator Reallocation." *Cambridge Quarterly of Healthcare Ethics*, 30(2), 272–284. doi:10.1017/S0963180120000833.] They argue that ventilators are "integrated technologies [that] are essential to one's functioning, not merely in acute situations, but across one's future life course, and they are part of one's relational narrative identity, and thus "taking away someone's ventilator is a direct assault on their bodily and social integrity."

7. See Department of Health and Human Services [Docket No.: HHS-OCR-2021–0004] RIN: 0945-AA15, 45 CFR Part 84, Discrimination on the Basis of Disability in Critical Health and Human Service Programs or Activities, p. 31; Agency: Office for Civil Rights (OCR), Office of the Secretary, HHS.

8. Specifically, they violate Americans with Disabilities Act of 1990 (ADA), 42 U.S.C. § 12101. They also violate Section 1557 of the Patient Protection and Affordable Care Act (ACA), 42 U.S.C. § 18116 and Section 504 of the Rehabilitation Act of 1973, 29 U.S.C. § 794.

9. K. Liddell, J. M. Skopek, S. Palmer, et al., "Who Gets the Ventilator? Important Legal Rights in a Pandemic," *Journal of Medical Ethics* 46 (2020): 421–26.

Chapter 6

Disability and Disproportionate Disadvantage

Kevin Timpe

INTRODUCTION

The COVID-19 pandemic has been bad. But it hasn't been equally bad for all. One of the ways in which it has been bad is that it has taken previously existing social inequalities and magnified them. Prior to the pandemic there were inequalities in economic security, access to quality healthcare, and educational opportunities, not to mention the inequalities forced on some people, given their identities, by structural racism, sexism, transphobia, ableism, xenophobia, and so on. One of the important effects of the pandemic is in terms of, as Carol Hay puts it, "exacerbating social problems that have always been there, making them such that even the socially privileged can no longer avoid them, and of course making them even worse for those who have been suffering their brunt all along."[1] Many of those groups that were already disadvantaged by social inequalities have been hit even harder by the pandemic. (This isn't a new phenomenon; it's been seen before with other catastrophic events, such as Hurricane Katrina.) Part of this is because the virus itself doesn't affect everyone equally. It's harder, on average, on older people than it is on younger people, on men than on women, and on Blacks than on whites. The subsequent shutdowns and economic uncertainty have, again on average, been more of a problem for poor and lower-middle-class people than on those who are wealthy or upper-middle class.

Some of these disparities have received significant public discussion. But another disproportional impact—namely, the fact that the pandemic has hit disabled individuals harder than nondisabled individuals—hasn't received quite as much public attention.[2] This claim, as with the earlier one, is a claim about average impact. Clearly, some nondisabled individuals have weathered the pandemic better than have some disabled individuals. But as a claim about how, on average, large groups of individuals have been affected, COVID has been harder on disabled populations. And this fact isn't as widely known or discussed as are some of the others. It'd be hard to not know that wealthy individuals with well-paying jobs and good insurance have had an easier time than hourly employees in service industries without employer-sponsored health insurance. In contrast, it's not as widely known that people with intellectual and developmental disabilities are three times more likely than nondisabled individuals to die if they are infected with COVID-19.[3] "The COVID-19 pandemic has highlighted systemic disadvantages that people with disabilities face in the health care system."[4] And that difference seems worth some attention, especially given that intellectually and developmentally disabled individuals are already disadvantaged in our society even apart from the pandemic. Looking at the patterns, bioethicists have concluded that disabled people are in "double jeopardy for marginalization in routine and preventive health care and, as demonstrated with COVID-19, in emergency preparedness and care."[5]

So in addition to all its impacts on public health, the economy, supply chains, and family dynamics, COVID has also highlighted many social inequalities that disabled individuals and families face. My goal in this chapter is to talk more about some of these inequalities. While acknowledging the full range of impacts on disabled individuals and families deserves attention, this chapter explores, at greater length, one particular kind of disproportionate impact: special education.[6] Don't get me wrong; virtually every student in the country has had their education affected by the pandemic. But, as we know, that impact isn't equal. To see how the pandemic has tended to impact those students who receive special education services harder, it'll be helpful to have a sense of how, in broad strokes, special education works in the United States. So that's the focus of the next section. The way that special education is done in public schools shaped how districts responded to the pandemic.

And then, in the final section, I look at how districts responded to the pandemic with respect to public education. What I hope to show is that how we've set up the structures of special education in the United States made our response to the pandemic worse, and not just for disabled students who receive special education. Many districts responded worse for all students given constraints related to special education. And this is telling. The fact that our public education system isn't set up to bear some of the pressures of a pandemic, or even other challenges like economic hardship, without harming students shows that the current system is problematic. I'm hoping that we can learn from the pandemic and take an opportunity to change our educational system in important ways. Because as much as we don't want to think about it yet, another challenge will come.

SPECIAL EDUCATION

The increased risk for marginalization isn't found only in the domain of public health. The pandemic has also revealed how public education is especially fragile for students with disabilities. Before turning to this, however, it will be helpful to have some background information regarding how public special education works in the United States.

The United Nations' 1975 Declaration on the Rights of Disabled Persons lists education among the human rights owed to disabled individuals. Their reasoning, in part, is that education is needed for full participation in social and civic life.[7] But historically, such a right was not often given. Most of our country's history hasn't included coordinated special education.

Massachusetts first required education in 1852. Mississippi became the last state to enact a compulsory public education law in 1918. Despite the move toward compulsory public education in general, it wasn't required for disabled students, and most states didn't even offer it. The Education for All Handicapped Children Act (EAHCA) became the first US federal law extending the right to public education to disabled students when it was enacted in 1975. Its passage was, in part, a response to a congressional investigation that found that less than half of the country's 8 million disabled children were receiving an appropriate education, and that nearly 25 percent weren't receiving any public education at all. The EAHCA was updated in 1990, becoming the Individuals with Disabilities Education Act (IDEA). IDEA guarantees disabled children the right to a "free appropriate public education" (FAPE). Furthermore, it requires that education to be provided in the "least restrictive environment" (LRE)—that is, for them to be educated with nondisabled students in the general education setting to the maximum extent appropriate. The purpose of the law is to prohibit a "separate but equal" approach to special education, since in our country's history separate never seems to be equal. IDEA specifically requires that

> each public [school] agency must ensure that: (i) to the maximum extent appropriate, children with disabilities, including children in public or private institutions or other care facilities, are educated with children who are nondisabled; and (ii) special classes, separate schooling, or other removal of children with disabilities from the regular educational environment occurs only if the nature

> or severity of the disability is such that education in regular classes with the use of supplementary aids and services cannot be achieved satisfactorily.

IDEA requires schools to develop an Individualized Education Plan (IEP) for all students with a qualifying disability. An IEP is a legal document describing how the school is going to provide any needed services or accommodations that will enable the disabled student to work toward appropriate goals and be involved in the general education curriculum. IEPs have to be reviewed and updated annually.

Public education in the United States is administered at the state rather than federal level. So IDEA isn't implemented by the federal Department of Education. Rather, each state develops its own application of IDEA. A state's special education program is then implemented through that state's local school districts. Each state also determines its own level and method of funding special education in public schools. As an "unfunded mandate," IDEA puts pressure on public schools and districts to provide services that are often costly. Budgetary concerns aren't allowed to restrict the services that are offered, but they often do in disguise. This means that the relationship between parents who think certain services are needed and school districts that don't have the money for them are often adversarial.

Given this general arrangement, when the pandemic hit during the spring of 2020, it was up to individual districts to implement their public education response to the pandemic. Unsurprisingly, district and state responses varied widely. Nevertheless, a number of patterns emerged. As we'll see in the next section, many of these responses were problematic, having negative impacts not only on disabled students but on all students. But the problems highlighted here don't capture all the challenges that different school across the country—and around the world—face. It's important to keep in mind that even under the best of conditions, special education remains problematic even though EAHCA and IDEA have been federal law for more than forty years. Schools have some incentive to follow IDEA's requirements, since failing to do so puts a district's federal and state education funding in jeopardy. But this sanction has never been enforced. So many districts do less than they're required to because they can get away with it. Our son's own district, for example, didn't even attempt to educate him in the general education classroom, bussing him past the neighborhood school across the street from our neighborhood to another school—that is, until we realized what the law required and pushed back.[8]

Evidence suggests our experience isn't unique. Many students who qualify for special education services under IDEA are not properly identified, especially in poorer communities. Forcing schools to follow the law often requires financial resources that many families do not have.[9] As a result, many children who should receive special education services "fall through the cracks," so to speak. Sometimes this is a result of a family not knowing how to navigate the procedures required. But many local and state educational services have policies in place that fail to provide what IDEA is supposed to guarantee. This suggests that perhaps a better metaphor is that students are actively "pushed into the cracks" if the district can get away with it.[10]

Consider, for example, Texas. In 2004 the Texas Education Agency (TEA) told its districts that they should aim for providing no more than 8.5 percent of their students with special education services. This was, they claimed, intended as a benchmark and not a cap, since such caps have no place under federal law. But upon investing, the US Department of Education's Office of Special Education Programs found that Texas districts had in fact used the 8.5 percent number as a cap, resulting in widespread denial of services required by IDEA. Providing special educational services to only 8.5 percent of students is nearly 35 percent below the rate of services provided in the other forty-nine states.[11] In 2018, the US Department of Education sent a letter to TEA that read as follows: "TEA's use of the 8.5 percent indicator contributed to a statewide pattern of practices that demonstrate that TEA did not ensure that all [districts] in the State properly identified, located and evaluated all children with disabilities who were in need of special education and related services."[12]

The Texas Education Agency would later admit that its policy led to up to 189,000 students who qualified for such services not receiving them. Governor Greg Abbott instructed TEA to prepare a plan to address those students who were denied services. While 101,400 students were eventually identified as eligible for compensatory services, as of May 2020 fewer than 8,000 of those students had actually received them.[13]

According to the most recent report by the US Department of Education, only twenty-one of the fifty states' educational services actually satisfy the requirements of IDEA.[14] More than five thousand written state complaints against schools or districts are filed under IDEA each year, and more than three times as many due process complaints.[15] While not every filed case indicates a failure for disabled individuals to receive the services afforded to them by IDEA, it's pretty obvious that that the law had not achieved the kind of protections it aims at, despite being over forty years old.

DISPROPORTIONATE DISADVANTAGE

This already bad situation of would get worse during the pandemic. The exact impact of the pandemic on education depends on specific educational policy and systems. Since special education in the United States is administered by individual districts, I look at a number of them in detail. However, many features of their response to the pandemic were shared by other districts. While my focus in on districts in the United States, similar issues arose in other countries. The *Guardian*, for example, reports of "'widespread failure' [in England] to restore special educational needs provision when children returned to school in September 2020."[16] Policy analysts in India note a similar, if not structurally worse, problem there:

> COVID 19 has brought unprecedented challenges in India one of which is its impact on school-going children and their regular education. While it is promising to see many thought pieces raising the issue and offering meaningful solutions to this issue, it is no surprise that we have yet again failed to recognize the highly excluded category of children with disabilities (CWDs) from the entire discourse. A staggering 75% of children with disabilities doesn't attend schools in India. When combined with other structural inequalities like poverty, caste, gender, religion etc., children with disabilities are more likely than other vulnerable categories to be excluded from education.[17]

These vulnerabilities can be found in a range of countries around the world.

Furthermore, it's also important to note that the impact of the pandemic wasn't felt equally by all disabled students. Students with less access to technology or with unreliable internet broadband were hit harder. Districts' and families' economic resources clearly mattered. In addition to economic and technology access concerns, the specific nature of students' disabilities played a role. A middle-class suburban student who uses a wheelchair may be able to access online learning resources as well as a nondisabled student, but the same won't be true for many students with intellectual disabilities even if they have the same economic resources. Given the financial impact that disabilities often have on families, there's no guarantee that a family's economic situation (and thus the public school system they have access to) will be insulated from disability status.

In the early days of the pandemic, many countries closed public schools in the face of the growing spread of the virus. More than 90 percent of students enrolled in preschool through higher education lost access to in-person education. While most countries closed schools at the federal level, the United States was one of only six countries that left that decision to more local levels of government.[18] The first US school district, Northshore School District near Seattle, shut down in-person instruction on March 5, 2020, initially shifting to instruction online. However, a week later it stopped providing instruction altogether, citing special education services and their inability to "meet the strict guidelines outlined in federal and state regulations."[19] This early move that would soon develop into a much wider pattern.

Schools received little guidance from the federal government's Department of Education, so they had to figure out how respond to the emerging situation at the state or district level. In New Jersey, of instance, state law prohibited providing special education services via telecommunications or other distance-learning tools. This limited their public schools' instructional options for disabled students in the early days of the pandemic. The New Jersey Board of Education relaxed those restrictions in early April 2020. Speaking on behalf of the board of education, assistant commissioner Peggy McDonald said that "the closure of schools during the COVID-19 pandemic has resulted in the need for the delivery of special-education instruction and related services . . . through alternative means. . . . Without this modification, students with disabilities would not be able to receive some of the services they are entitled to."[20] This was a particular concern give that the Newark Public School District, the state's largest public district, had been found guilty of failing to enforce special education law in 2019, resulting in a state order to take corrective action. (Fourteen other New Jersey districts also failed to meet four or more of the nine requirements stemming from an earlier lawsuit against seventy-six districts in the state.)[21] But numerous parents denied that their children were given the services they qualified for during the early transition.[22]

Other states preemptively made decisions in an effort to avoid legal trouble. Natalia Alamdari reported that "Delaware public school districts have balked at the idea of remote learning [in their spring 2020 response to the pandemic] out of fear of being sued, especially related to meeting the needs of special education students."[23] The majority of lawsuits over special education services settle out of court, costing the districts significant amounts of money. According to Alamdari, some Delaware districts instructed their teachers to not offer any official instruction during the first few weeks of the pandemic to avoid opening themselves up to such lawsuits. Other districts, including Jefferson County Public Schools, the largest public school district in Kentucky, admitted that concerns about equity led them to not move official instruction online.[24]

According to a white paper from Meira Levinson at Harvard's Edmond J. Safra Center for Ethics, many states and districts decided to "to level down to offer no educational services to anyone rather than violate principles of equity as policy-makers understood them."[25] Public schools were aware that official instructional time offered remotely through distance learning would have to be a full replacement for face-to-face instruction, thus requiring schools to "abide by all IEPs, 504s, and other instructional needs of students."[26] But some services required by students' IEPs can't be provided remotely. If a school district was offering official instruction online and couldn't provide all IEP services remotely, then it would be in violation of state and federal law and potentially guilty of discriminating against disabled students. By mid-March, an increasing number of public schools had announced that they were "canceling all government-mandated meetings for special-needs students until schools reopen—which might not be until fall [of 2020]."[27]

The federal Department of Education, led by then Secretary of Education Betsy DeVos, tried to counter this trend. The department admitted that "if an LEA [local education agency] closes its schools to slow or stop the spread of spread of COVID-19, and does not provide any educational services to the general student population, then an LEA would not be required to provide services to students with disabilities during that same period."[28] But the Department of Education's Office of Special Education and Rehabilitative Services advised in mid-March that

> to be clear: ensuring compliance with the Individuals with Disabilities Education Act (IDEA), Section 504 of the Rehabilitation Act (Section 504), and Title II of the Americans with Disabilities Act *should not prevent any school from offering educational programs through distance instruction*. . . . [Districts] should not opt to close or decline to provide distance instruction, at the expense of students, to address matters pertaining to services for students with disabilities.[29]

Within days of the above guidance from the education department, the American Association of School Superintendents cautioned that

> it's one thing for ED [the US Department of Education] to understand this but another for Courts to understand this is the case. The law is still the law, and ED's suggestion that districts are responsible for "still meet[ing] their legal obligations by providing children with disabilities equally effective alternate access to the curriculum or services provided to other students" will be an insurmountable challenge for some districts.[30]

Their hesitancy and concern about legal ramifications makes sense, especially since the federal government also reminded schools that "if the school is open and serving other students, the school must ensure that the student continues to receive a free appropriate public education (FAPE)."[31] But the federal government also instructed schools that "if a school district closes its schools and does not provide any educational services to the general student population, then a school would not be required to provide services to students with disabilities during that same period of time."[32] Some districts took this as a way to avoid the need to comply with IDEA's demands.

In April 2020, DeVos announced that the education department would not provide waivers "for any of the core tenets of the IDEA or Section 504 of the Rehabilitation Act of 1973, most notably a free appropriate public education (FAPE) in the least restrictive environment (LRE)."[33] Overall, it is hard to see the administration's response as little more than doublespeak, requiring of schools what the administration in no way equipped them to provide. It's not surprising then that the vast majority of districts closed not only their buildings but also their official instructional offerings through the end of the school year.[34]

Let's look more closely at how one district, Grand Rapids Public Schools (GRPS), a public school district in Michigan, responded to this situation. Like all schools in Michigan, GRPS was initially closed on March 16, 2020, by an executive order from Governor Gretchen Whitmer.[35] GRPS's legal counsel confirmed to district administrators that "if a school chooses to use virtual instruction in place of in-person instruction for general education students during the closure, the school *must* ensure equal access for *all* students and FAPE for students with disabilities."[36] This would involve districts needing to provide all related services—occupational therapy, physical therapy, speech therapy, psychological services, social work services, nursing services, and so on—remotely as well. The same day the district received this confirmation from its legal counsel, GRPS executive director of special education and early intervention services Laura LaMore wrote in an e-mail:

> No official instruction? No FAPE. When we shift from [Optional Online Enrichment] Resources to [official] Instruction, we shift to FAPE If we move to a virtual learning platform, we will be mandated to open every IEP (2843), 504 Plan (188) and NPSP [non-public service plan] (294)—and at least amend . . . to identify what they will be receiving as our offer of FAPE. (Because FAPE needs to change when environment changes. . . .) We will be crushed with compliance when we should be thinking about instruction.[37]

But the need to provide FAPE to disabled students could be avoided simply by not providing any educational services to the general student population. LaMore described this realization as "a game changer."[38]

Whitmer issued an executive order on April 2, 2020, suspending in-person instruction and closing school buildings to the public for the remainder of the school year.[39] That executive order also required each public school district to implement a Continuity of Learning Plan (also known as a Distance Learning Plan) by April 28. While this executive order effectively allowed districts to offer no more official instruction for the rest of the school year, nothing in the order prohibited schools from providing instruction. That is, districts could continue to offer official instruction through electronic or virtual means, but doing so would, as already indicated, require that they live up to the requirements of IDEA.

GRPS's Continuity of Learning Plan, the COVID-19 response plan required by Whitmer's executive order, was "the district's approach to providing high-quality academic, social-emotional, and wellness support for students and families throughout the school closures during Spring 2020."[40] It claimed to be "universally designed to be inclusive across all grade levels"[41] for all students, including those receiving special education services. But in order to not need to follow the requirements of IDEA in providing FAPE, the Continuity of Learning Plan consisted entirely of optional resources and supplemental learning. This would enable the district to focus on delivering educational opportunities to students "and not compliance"[42] with state and federal laws requiring equity of access for disabled students.

Our son was among those who then didn't receive all the therapies that were supposed to be provided by GRPS as part of their public education services. While there was an attempt to offer some of these services remotely as part of the "optional resources and supplemental learning" resources, they just couldn't replace what he usually received.

The denial of educational opportunities and services, and the resulting leveling down of education based on the recognition that special education law couldn't be followed, wasn't the only disproportionate disadvantage faced by disabled students in public school districts. In at least some cases, transition documents such as distance learning surveys were not available in alternative format for blind students or parents. Nor were they available in translation for English as a second language families, many of whom also have disabilities.[43] Many of the assistive technologies students rely on to access their nature were not compatible with the online platforms many districts turned to. A blind student, for example, would not be able to access tactile maps via Zoom.[44] While all the online technologies, platforms, and apps districts used were required to comply with federal and state guidelines for the visually impaired, this requirement was often ignored. As one parent put it, "[There are] students who rely on structure their new virtual classrooms can't provide; dyslexic or reading-delayed students who have to read even more in order to access online learning."[45]

Children who receive special education are sometimes afforded Extended School Year (ESY) services to protect against regression during the summer months. According to the Department of Education, "a child's entitlement to needed ESY services continues to apply even if schools and other facilities are closed due to COVID-19."[46] But many districts did not provide such services at all during the summer of 2020. The Department of Education also indicated that "districts shall, to the extent practicable and necessary, make individualized determinations whether and to what extent compensatory services may be needed for pupils after the school closure period prompted by the COVID-19 state of emergency and/or state of disaster ends."[47] As of this writing, that has not happened in many districts. The situation mentioned earlier involving the Texas Education Agency, so far the only large-scale effort to provide compensatory services, indicates that the process of seeking to evaluate for and provide compensatory services is likely to be a massive failure. Even for those disabled students who are able to secure such services, receiving them will often require additional work by their families. As Lisa Flores, whose son attends a Texas public school, puts it, "The onus is still on parents to ask for compensatory services, and it will still be on parents once this is over. . . . I doubt any district will preemptively offer compensatory education. They will stay quiet and only consider it if a parent brings it up."[48] As with other aspects of special education, the burden too often falls to families to make sure districts follow through.

As problematic as this is, there were other disproportionate effects on families of disabled students. Just as many families with health concerns felt a greater need to take precautions in an attempt to avoid being infected, so too did many families with disabled members. Online education often requires substantially more involvement from parents of disabled students who otherwise require an aide or paraprofessional to access their education. Either my spouse or I had to be on Zoom with our son for every aspect of his online schooling, often while trying to also assist our other two children and finding time to teach my own classes at my university. Parents, even involved ones, are not professionally trained therapists or educators. Even if they have the time and flexibility to devote to their children's needs (which, to be quite frank, many of them didn't), they cannot provide the highly specific and intensive supports that disabilities sometimes require: "There are students with physical disabilities who receive therapies their parents aren't trained to do; students with attention issues who find it difficult to focus in a classroom, let alone on video instruction."[49]

Having to cancel those services due to public health concerns means that many of those students were less prepared, both compared to nonpandemic years but also compared to their nondisabled peers who don't need such services, when schools reopened in the fall of 2020. One survey in the UK reported that 69 percent of families with children with learning disabilities reported having their social services cut the first half of 2020.[50] As Ami Harbin and Alice MacLachlan put it, the pandemic has called into question "the assumed self-sufficiently of the nuclear family."[51]

The impact of the pandemic, of course, didn't end with the 2019–2020 school year. Most schools would reopen to instruction in the fall of 2020, though often virtually. Many of the increased demands on working parents and families would return. But as we've seen, these demands are not uniform, and disabled families continue to bear a larger share of them. In September 2020, the federal Office of Special Education Programs reminded state and local education agencies that "no matter what primary instructional delivery approach is chosen, SEAs [state education agencies], LEAs [local education agencies], and individualized education program (IEP) Teams remain responsible for ensuring that a free appropriate public education (FAPE) is provided to all children with disabilities."[52] Some school districts, however, sought to use educational funds designated for special education services to pay for "non–special education duties such as check-in duties, temperature taking, covering classes, etc.," forcing state departments of education to note that "any non–special education duties must be paid from funds other than special education, and may not be reimbursed with state special education categorical aid."[53] Though already underfunded, special education programs were seen as a source of funding for other pandemic-related services.

CONCLUSION

The pandemic, as Julia Watts Belser puts it, "hits hardest among communities that are already marginalized."[54] IDEA was developed to provide for the education of previous marginalized individuals. But IDEA is an unfunded mandate, putting obligations on public school districts without providing funding for those obligations. It's understandable, then, that districts would be motivated by a concern for cost—both of providing services and for the lawsuits they were afraid of. But as the Supreme Court decided in *Goldberg v. Kelly*, the state's interest in the general welfare and education of its citizens "clearly outweighs" its concern "to prevent any increase in its fiscal and administrative burdens. . . . Public assistance, then, is not mere charity, but a means to 'promote the general Welfare, and secure the Blessings of Liberty to ourselves and all our Posterity.'"[55] The purpose of special education in the United States is provide "a more equitable allocation of resources [that] is essential for the Federal Government to meet its responsibility to provide an equal educational opportunity for all individuals"[56] As we've seen, however, concerns about living up to the law led school districts to choose not to provide education to *any* student.

Public health threats like COVID require a structural response. It's not enough for individuals to make personal choices they think are best for them. We need public health policy, guidance, and coordination. In a similar way, the ability of a country or state to provide special education requires a good structural response. While public special education is governed by federal law, the pandemic has magnified many of the previously existing structural inequalities that already existed in how the United States approaches special education. While the pandemic has been felt by all, its harms have not been uniform. And those harms have often fallen disproportionately on those who are least able to bear them.[57]

BIBLIOGRAPHY

Adams, Richard. "Pupils with Special Needs 'Forgotten' as English Schools Reopen." *Guardian*, September 4, 2020. https://www.theguardian.com/education/2020/sep/04/special-needs-pupils-forgotten-english-schools-reopen.

Alamdari, Natalia. "Delaware Public Schools Are Beginning Remote Learning. But Should They Fear Future Lawsuits?" *Delaware Online*, April 1, 2020. https://www.delawareonline.com/story/news/2020/04/01/coronavirus-should-delaware-schools-fear-lawsuits-remote-learning-begins/5094015002/.

American Association of School Superintendents. "ED Issues Guidance on FAPE During COVID-19." 2020. https://web.archive.org/web/20210917042059/https:/www.aasa.org/policy-blogs.aspx?id=44560&blogid=84002

Artiga, Samantha, Rachel Garfield, and Kendal Orgera. 2020. "Communities of Color at Higher Risk for Health and Economic Challenges due to COVID-19." Kaiser Family Foundation, April 7, 2020. https://www.kff.org/coronavirus-covid-19/issue-brief/communities-of-color-at-higher-risk-for-health-and-economic-challenges-due-to-covid-19/.

Autistic Self Advocacy Network. "Evaluation Framework for Crisis Standard of Care," April 9, 2020. https://autisticadvocacy.org/wp-content/uploads/2020/04/Evaluation-framework-for-crisis-standards-of-care-plans-4.9.20-final.pdf.

Bagchi, Suparna, Josephine Mak, Qunna Li, Edward Sheriff, Elisabeth Mungai, Angela Anttila, Minn Minn Soe, Jonathan R. Edwards, Andrea L. Benin, Daniel A. Pollock, et al. "Rates of COVID-19 among Residents and Staff Members in Nursing Homes—United States, May 25–November 22, 2020." Centers for Disease Control and Prevention. https://www.cdc.gov/mmwr/volumes/70/wr/mm7002e2.htm.

Ballantyne, Angela. "ICU Triage: How Many Lives or Whose Lives?" *Journal of Medical Ethics Blog*, April 7, 2020, https://blogs.bmj.com/medical-ethics/2020/04/07/icu-triage-how-many-lives-or-whose-lives/.

Bennett, Jana M. 2020. "Disabilities in Hiding: How the Pandemic Might Shape Justice for All of Us." *Berkley Forum: Religion and the COVID-19 Pandemic: Vulnerable Populations*, April 16, 2020. https://berkleycenter.georgetown.edu/responses/disabilities-in-hiding-how-the-pandemic-might-shape-justice-for-all-of-us.

Bose, Devna. "As Newark Moves to Virtual Learning, Special Education is an Especially 'Heavy Lift.'" *Chalkbeat Newark*, April 15, 2020. https://newark.chalkbeat.org/2020/4/15/21225553/as-newark-moves-to-virtual-learning-special-education-is-an-especially-heavy-lift.

Belser, Julia Watts. "Disability and the Politics of Vulnerability." *Berkley Forum: Religion and the COVID-19 Pandemic: Vulnerable Populations*, April 15, 2020. https://berkleycenter.georgetown.edu/responses/disability-and-the-politics-of-vulnerability.

Boulicaulty, Marion, and Sarah S. Richardson. "Analyzing COVID-19 Sex Difference Claims: The Harvard GenderSci Lab." *APA Newsletter on Feminism and Philosophy* 20, no. 1 (2020): 3–7.

Burckhardt, Holger, and Bennett Jäger. "On Human Rights and Human Duties: Is There a Moral Obligation to Inclusion?" 68–73. In *Human Rights and Disability: Interdisciplinary Perspectives*, ed. John-Steward Gordan, Johann-Christian Poker, and Holger Burckhart. New York: Routledge, 2017.

Center for Appropriate Dispute Resolution in Special Education. *IDEA Data Brief: Written State Complaints*. September 2017. https://www.cadreworks.org/sites/default/files/resources/WSC%20Brief_WebFinal_9.2017.pdf.

Centers for Disease Control and Prevention. "Preparing for COVID-19 in Nursing Homes." 2020. https://www.cdc.gov/coronavirus/2019-ncov/hcp/long-term-care.html.

Chung, Nicole. "My Child Has a Disability. What Will Her Education Be Like This Year?" *New York Times*, September 10, 2020. https://www.nytimes.com/interactive/2020/09/10/magazine/special-education-covid.html.

DeVos, Betsy. "Recommended Waiver Authority Under Section 3511(d)(4) of Division A of the Coronavirus Aid, Relief, and Economic Security Act ('CARES Act)." US Department of Education, April 27, 2020. https://www2.ed.gov/documents/coronavirus/cares-waiver-report.pdf

Down Syndrome Prenatal Testing. "Coronavirus: Sixteen Times More Lethal for Kids with Intellectual Disabilities." 2020. http://www.downsyndromeprenataltesting.com/coronavirus-sixteen-times-more-lethal-for-kids-with-intellectual-disabilities/.

Ellis, Blake, and Melanie Hicken. "Covid-19 Is Ravaging Nursing Homes. Government Records Show Why." CNN, April 24, 2020. https://www.cnn.com/2020/04/24/us/nursing-homes-coronavirus-invs/index.html.

FAIRHealth. "Risk Factors for COVID-19 Mortality among Privately Insured Patients." 2020. https://s3.amazonaws.com/media2.fairhealth.org/whitepaper/asset/Risk%20Factors%20for%20COVID-19%20Mortality%20among%20Privately%20Insured%20Patients%20-%20A%20Claims%20Data%20Analysis%20-%20A%20FAIR%20Health%20White%20Paper.pdf. https://s3.amazonaws.com/media2.fairhealth.org/whitepaper/asset/Risk%20Factors%20for%20COVID-19%20Mortality%20among%20Privately%20Insured%20Patients%20-%20A%20Claims%20Data%20Analysis%20-%20A%20FAIR%20Health%20White%20Paper.pdf

Fischer, Max, and Emma Bubolo. "As Coronavirus Deepens Inequality, Inequality Worsens Its Spread." *New York Times*, March 15, 2020. https://www.nytimes.com/2020/03/15/world/europe/coronavirus-inequality.html.

Garg, Shikha, Lindsay Kim, Michael Whitaker, Alissa O'Halloran, Charisse Cummings, Rachel Holstein, Mila Prill, Shua J. Chai, Pam D. Kirley, Nisha B. Alden, et al. "Hospitalization Rates and Characteristics of Patients Hospitalized with Laboratory-Confirmed Coronavirus Disease 2019—COVID-NET, 14 States, March 1–30, 2020." *Morbidity and Mortality Weekly Report* 69, no. 15 (2020): 458–464.

Goldberg, Daniel S. "Structural Stigma, Legal Epidemiology, and COVID-19: The Ethical Imperative to Act Upstream." *Kennedy Institute of Ethics Journal*, June 17, 2020. https://kiej.georgetown.edu/structural-stigma-covid-19-special-issue/.

Guidry-Grimes, Laura, Katie Savin, Joseph A. Stramondo, Joel Michael Reynolds, Marina Tsaplina, Teresa Blankmeyer Burke, Angela Ballantyne, Eva Feder Kittay, Devan Stahl, Jackie Leach Scully, et al. "Disability Rights as a Necessary Framework for Crisis Standards of Care and the Future of Healthcare." *Hastings Center Report* 50, no. 3 (May/June 2020): 28–32. https://onlinelibrary.wiley.com/doi/abs/10.1002/hast.1128.

Harbin, Ami, and Alice MacLachlan. "Pandemic Parenting." *APA Newsletter on Feminism and Philosophy* 20, no. 1 (2020): 22–26.

Harris, Edel. "Lockdown Has Brought Families of Learning Disabled People to Their Knees." *Guardian*, August 11, 2020. https://www.theguardian.com/society/2020/aug/11/lockdown-families-learning-disabled-people-coronavirus.

Hawkins, R. B., E. J. Charles, and J. H. Mehaffey. "Socio-economic Status and COVID-19-Related Cases and Fatalities." *Public Health* 189 (2020): 129–34.

Hay, Carol. "How Privilege Structures Pandemic Narratives." *APA Newsletter on Feminism* 20, no. 1 (2020): 7–12.

Hill, Faith. "The Pandemic Is a Crisis for Students with Special Needs." *Atlantic*, April 18, 2020. https://www.theatlantic.com/education/archive/2020/04/special-education-goes-remote-covid-19-pandemic/610231/.

Kansas State Department of Education. "School Year 2020–21 Compliance with the Individuals with Disabilties Education Act and the Kansas Special Education for Exceptional Children Act for Reopening Schools During the COVID-19 Pandemic." April 1, 2021. https://www.ksde.org/Portals/0/ECSETS/Announcements/COVID-SpEd-FAQ.pdf.

Kittay, Eva Feder. "People with Disabilities Are at a Disadvantage When Scarce Medical Resources Are Being Allocated." *STAT News*, April 29, 2020. https://www.statnews.com/2020/04/29/people-disabilities-disadvantage-covid-19-scarce-medical-resources/.

Leamanczyk, Lauren. "KARE 11 Investigates: Special Needs Students Left without Distance Learning Help." KARE 11, September 24, 2020. https://www.kare11.com/article/news/investigations/kare-11-investigates-special-needs-students-left-without-distance-learning-help/89-a82ebc79-e809-4884-995b-21cd10fe1453.

Levine, Hallie. "As the Country Opens Up, Children with Disabilities are Getting Left Behind." *New York Times*, June 10, 2020. https://www.nytimes.com/2020/06/10/parenting/coronavirus-children-disabilities.html.

Levinson, Meira. *Educational Ethics during a Pandemic*. Edmond J. Safra Center for Ethics at Harvard University. May 16, 2020. https://ethics.harvard.edu/files/center-for-ethics/files/17educationalethics2.pdf.

Matos, Alejandra. "'Delayed or Denied': Feds Find Texas Schools Violated Special Education Laws." *Houston Chronicle*, January 10, 2018. https://www.chron.com/politics/texas/article/Delayed-or-denied-Feds-finds-Texas-schools-12489083.php.

Mitchell, Damon. "Families of Students with Disabilities Are Feeling Left out of Nashville's Plan for Virtual Learning." WPLN Nashville Public Radio, August 20, 2020. https://wpln.org/post/families-of-students-with-disabilities-are-feeling-left-out-of-nashvilles-plan-for-virtual-learning/.

Mooney, John. "Meeting Remotely, State BOE OKs Remote Learning for Special-Needs Students." *NJ Spotlight News*, April 2, 2020. https://www.njspotlight.com/2020/04/meeting-remotely-state-boe-oks-remote-learning-for-special-needs-students/.

Nelson, Ryan H., and Leslie P. Francis. "Intellectual Disability and Justice in a Pandemic." *Kennedy Institute of Ethics Journal*, June 17, 2020. https://kiej.georgetown.edu/intellectual-disability-pandemic-special-issue/.

Northshore School District. "Letter to Families: Gov. Inslee's Announcement." March 12, 2020. https://www.nsd.org/blog/~board/superintendent-blog/post/letter-to-families-gov-inslees-announcement.

Nussbaum, Martha. "The Capabilities of People with Cognitive Disabilities," 75–95. In *Cognitive Diasbility and Its Challenge to Moral Philosophy*, ed. Eva Feder Kittay and Licia Carlson. Malden, MA: Wiley-Blackwell, 2010.

Pandey, Pooja, and Sumyesh Srivastava. "Excluding the Excluded: India's Response to the Education of Children with Disabilities During Covid-19." *Times of India*, April 26, 2020. https://timesofindia.indiatimes.com/blogs/voices/excluding-the-excluded-indias-response-to-the-education-of-children-with-disabilities-during-covid-19/.

Partnership for Inclusive Disaster Strategies. "National Call to Action." March 3, 2020. https://mailchi.mp/disasterstrategies/covid19-disability-rights-call-to-action-with-org-support.

Pasachoff, Eloise. "Special Education, Poverty, and the Limits of Private Enforcement." *Notre Dame Law Review* 86, no. 4 (2011): 1413–94.

Pascoe, Jordan, and Mitch Stripling. "Surging Solidarity: Reorienting Ethics for Pandemics." *Kennedy Institute of Ethics Journal*, June 17, 2020. https://kiej.georgetown.edu/surging-solidarity-special-issue/.

Rabin, Roni Caryn. "Developmental Disabilities Heighten Risk of Covid Death." *New York Times*, November 11, 2020. https://www.nytimes.com/2020/11/10/health/covid-developmental-disabilities.html.

Ratner, Todd. "A Matter of Civil Rights." Ratner Law. April 4, 2016. https://ratnerplc.com/a-matter-of-civil-rights/.

Richards, Erin. "Is Online School Illegal? With Schools Closing from Coronavirus, Special Education Concerns Give Districts Pause." *USA Today*, March 19, 2020. https://www.usatoday.com/story/news/education/2020/03/19/coronavirus-online-school-closing-special-education-teacher-distance-learning/2863503001/.

Sabatello, May, Teresa Blankmeyer Burke, Katherine E. McDonald, and Paul S. Appelbaum. "Disability, Ethics, and Health Care in the COVID-19 Pandemic." *Public Health Ethics* 110, no. 10 (2020): 1523–27.

Savin, Katie, and Luara Guidy-Grimes. "Confronting Disability Discrimination during the Pandemic." Hastings Center, April 2, 2020. https://www.thehastingscenter.org/confronting-disability-discrimination-during-the-pandemic/.

Scully, Jackie Leach. "Disablism in a Time of Pandemic: Some Things Don't Change." *International Journal of Feminist Approaches to Bioethics Blog*, April 1, 2020. https://www.ijfab.org/blog/2020/04/disablism-in-a-time-of-pandemic-some-things-dont-change/.

Stramondo, Joseph. "COVID-19 Triage and Disability: What NOT To Do." *Bioethics Today*, March 30, 2020. https://www.bioethics.net/2020/03/covid-19-triage-and-disability-what-not-to-do/.

"The Striking Racial Divide in How Covid-19 Has Hit Nursing Homes." *New York Times*, May 21, 2020. https://www.nytimes.com/article/coronavirus-nursing-homes-racial-disparity.html.

Timpe, Kevin. *Disability and Inclusive Communities*. Grand Rapids, MI: Calvin University Press, 2018.

———. "What Are Intended as Systems of Support Become Systems of Struggle." *Ought: The Journal of Autistic Culture* 3.1 (2021), 38 –50.

Turk, Margaret A., Scott D. Landes, Margaret K. Formica, and Katherine D. Goss. "Intellectual and Developmental Disability and COVID-19 Case-fatality Trends: TriNexT Analysis." *Disability Health Journal* 13, no. 3 (2020): 100942. https://www.ncbi.nlm.nih.gov/pmc/articles/PMC7245650/.

UK Office for National Statistics. "Updated Estimates of Coronavirus (COVID-19) Related Deaths by Disability Status, England 24 January to 20 November 2020." February 11, 2021. https://www.ons.gov.uk/peoplepopulationandcommunity/birthsdeathsandmarriages/deaths/articles/coronaviruscovid19relateddeathsbydisabilitystatusenglandandwales/24januaryto20november2020.

United Nations. "Declaration on the Rights of Disabled Persons." 1975. https://www.ohchr.org/EN/ProfessionalInterest/Pages/RightsOfDisabledPersons.aspx.

United States Courts. "Just the Facts: Americans with Disabilities Act." July 12, 2018. https://www.uscourts.gov/news/2018/07/12/just-facts-americans-disabilities-act.

US Department of Education. "2020 Determination Letters on State Implementation of IDEA." 2020. https://sites.ed.gov/idea/files/ideafactsheet-determinations-2020.pdf.

———. "Questions and Answers on Providing Services to Children with Disabilities during the Coronavirus Disease 2019 Outbreak (March 2020)." 2020. https://sites.ed.gov/idea/idea-files/q-and-a-providing-services-to-children-with-disabilities-during-the-coronavirus-disease-2019-outbreak/.

———. "Supplemental Fact Sheet: Addressing the Risk of COVID-19 in Preschool, Elementary and Secondary Schools While Serving Children with Disabilities." March 21, 2020. https://www2.ed.gov/about/offices/list/ocr/frontpage/faq/rr/policyguidance/Supple%20Fact%20Sheet%203.21.20%20FINAL.pdf.

US Department of Education, Office for Civil Rights. "Fact Sheet: Addressing the Risk of COVID-19 in Schools While Protecting the Civil Rights of Students," March 16, 2020. https://www2.ed.gov/about/offices/list/ocr/docs/ocr-coronavirus-fact-sheet.pdf.

US Department of Education, Office of Special Education Programs. "OSEP QA 20–01." September 28, 2020. https://sites.ed.gov/idea/files/qa-provision-of-services-idea-part-b-09-28-2020.pdf.

Valles, Sean A. "The Predictable Inequities of COVID-19 in the US: Fundamental Causes and Broken Assumptions." *Kennedy Institute of Ethics Journal*, June 17, 2020. https://kiej.georgetown.edu/predictable-inequities-covid-19-special-issue/.

Vu, Minh, Kristina Laney, and Susan Ryan. "2019 was Another Record-Breaking Year for Federal ADA Title III Lawsuits." *ADA Title III News & Insights*, February 20, 2020. https://www.adatitleiii.com/2020/02/2019-was-another-record-breaking-year-for-federal-ada-title-iii-lawsuits/.

Wadman, Meredith. "COVID-19 Is 10 Times Deadlier for People with Down Syndrome, Raising Calls for Early Vaccination." *Science*, December 15, 2020. https://www.sciencemag.org/news/2020/12/covid-19-10-times-deadlier-people-down-syndrome-raising-calls-early-vaccination.

Wall, Patrick, and Devna Bose. "Newark Fails to Enforce Key Special Education Mandates, State Report Says." *Chalkbeat Newark*, November 25, 2019. https://newark.chalkbeat.org/2019/11/25/21109348/newark-fails-to-enforce-key-special-education-mandates-state-report-says.

Weale, Sally. "English Schools 'Using Coronavirus as Excuse' Not to Teach Special Education Pupils." *Guardian*, July 1, 2020. https://www.theguardian.com/education/2020/jul/01/english-schools-using-coronavirus-as-excuse-not-to-teach-special-needs-pupils.

———. "Special Needs Pupils in England 'Pushed to One Side' in Covid Crisis." *Guardian*, February 19, 2021. https: //www.theguardian.com/education/2021/feb/19/special-needs-pupils-in-england-pushed-to-one-side-in-covid-crisis.

Webb, Shelby. "Lost Time: Many Texas Special Education Students Say They Are Still Waiting for Help to Make Up for Delays and Denials." *Houston Chronicle*, May 7, 2020. https://www.houstonchronicle.com/news/investigations/article/federal-law-students-denied-special-education-15253514.php.

NOTES

1. Carol Hay, "How Privilege Structures Pandemic Narratives," *APA Newsletter on Feminism* 20, no. 1 (2020): 8.

2. There has been some discussion. For worthwhile discussions, see Laura Guidry-Grimes, Katie Savin, Joseph A. Stramondo, Joel Michael Reynolds, Marina Tsaplina, Teresa Blankmeyer Burke, Angela Ballantyne, Eva Feder Kittay, Devan Stahl, Jackie Leach Scully, et al., "Disability Rights as a Necessary Framework for Crisis Standards of Care and the Future of Healthcare," *Hastings Center Report* 50, no. 3 (May/June 2020): 28–32, https://onlinelibrary.wiley.com/doi/abs/10.1002/hast.1128; Julia Watts Belser, "Disability and the Politics of Vulnerability," *Berkley Forum: Religion and the COVID-19 Pandemic: Vulnerable Populations*, April 15, 2020, https://berkleycenter.georgetown.edu/responses/disability-and-the-politics-of-vulnerability; Meredith Wadman, "COVID-19 Is 10 Times Deadlier for People with Down Syndrome, Raising Calls for Early Vaccination," *Science*, December 15, 2020, https://www.sciencemag.org/news/2020/12/covid-19-10-times-deadlier-people-down-syndrome-raising-calls-early-vaccination; Margaret A. Turk, Scott D. Landes, Margaret K. Formica, and Katherine D. Goss, "Intellectual and Developmental Disability and COVID-19 Case-fatality Trends: TriNexT Analysis," *Disability Health Journal* 13, no. 3 (2020): 100942, https://www.ncbi.nlm.nih.gov/pmc/articles/PMC7245650/; UK Office for

National Statistics, "Updated Estimates of Coronavirus (COVID-19) Related Deaths by Disability Status, England 24 January to 20 November 2020," February 11, 2021, https://www.ons.gov.uk/peoplepopulationandcommunity/birthsdeathsandmarriages/deaths/articles/coronaviruscovid19relateddeathsbydisabilitystatusenglandandwales/24januaryto20november2020; and Down Syndrome Prenatal Testing, "Coronavirus: Sixteen Times More Lethal for Kids with Intellectual Disabilities," 2020, http://www.downsyndromeprenataltesting.com/coronavirus-sixteen-times-more-lethal-for-kids-with-intellectual-disabilities/.

3. Roni Caryn Rabin, "Developmental Disabilities Heighten Risk of Covid Death," *New York Times*, November 11, 2020, https: //www.nytimes.com/2020/11/10/health/covid-developmental-disabilities.html.

4. Guidry-Grimes et al., "Disability Rights as a Necessary Framework."

5. May Sabatello, Teresa Blankmeyer Burke, Katherine E. McDonald, and Paul S. Appelbaum, "Disability, Ethics, and Health Care in the COVID-19 Pandemic," *Public Health Ethics* 110, no. 10 (2020): 1523 (footnotes omitted).

6. I find the phrase "special education" to be problematic, for similar reasons to why many individuals involved with disability studies or disability rights think the phrase "special needs" is problematic. While the testimony of individuals with disabilities isn't uniform with respect to a number of terminological issues, many object to the use of "special needs" and "special education" in a way we ought to take seriously. Furthermore, it is not the aim or importance of education that is "special"; rather it is primarily the delivery modalities of that education that is special. Thinking of "special education" as distinct from just plain education makes it too easy to apply different standards, thereby contributing to discrimination or ableism. Nevertheless, "special education" is the leading term in the relevant subsection of education literature and is a term with specific legal force (see, e.g., IDEA 300.39). Given this, I'll use the term but with reservations.

7. United Nations, "Declaration on the Rights of Disabled Persons," 1975, https://www.ohchr.org/EN/ProfessionalInterest/Pages/RightsOfDisabledPersons.aspx. See also the discussion in Holger Burckhardt and Bennett Jäger, "On Human Rights and Human Duties: Is There a Moral Obligation to Inclusion?" 68–73, in *Human Rights and Disability: Interdisciplinary Perspectives*, ed. John-Steward Gordan, Johann-Christian Poker, and Holger Burckhart (New York: Routledge, 2017).

8. A fuller account of this story can be found in Kevin Timpe, *Disability and Inclusive Communities* (Grand Rapids, MI: Calvin University Press, 2018), chap. 1.

9. Eloise Pasachoff writes that "the available evidence suggests that wealthier parents continue to come out ahead in the enforcement game. At the individual and intra-district level, the evidence is largely anecdotal, but it is consistent and widespread. Throughout the country, scholars and commentators provide repeated examples of parents with greater financial resources disproportionately taking advantage of the IDEA's private enforcement mechanisms in comparison to their less well-heeled neighbors. . . . Our findings are consistent with the idea that families with more financial (and perhaps also educational) resources are better situated to pursue their rights under the IDEA" (Eloise Pasachoff, "Special Education, Poverty, and the Limits of Private Enforcement," *Notre Dame Law Review* 86, no. 4 (2011): 1426f).

10. For more on related issues, see Kevin Timpe, "What Are Intended as Systems of Support become Systems of Struggle," *Ought: The Journal of Autistic Culture*.

11. Nicole Chung, "My Child Has a Disability. What Will Her Education Be Like This Year?" *New York Times*, September 10, 2020, https://www.nytimes.com/interactive/2020/09/10/magazine/special-education-covid.html.

12. Alejandra Matos, "'Delayed or Denied': Feds Find Texas Schools Violated Special Education Laws," *Houston Chronicle*, January 10, 2018, https://www.chron.com/politics/texas/article/Delayed-or-denied-Feds-finds-Texas-schools-12489083.php.

13. Shelby Webb, "Lost Time: Many Texas Special Education Students Say They Are Still Waiting for Help to Make Up for Delays and Denials," *Houston Chronicle*, May 7, 2020, https://www.houstonchronicle.com/news/investigations/article/federal-law-students-denied-special-education-15253514.php.

14. US Department of Education, "2020 Determination Letters on State Implementation of IDEA," 2020. https://sites.ed.gov/idea/files/ideafactsheet-determinations-2020.pdf. The report also tracks ten other localities in addition to states (e.g., the District of Columbia, the Bureau of Indian Education, and associated states such as American Samoa, Guam, and Puerto Rico); of these, only one was found to meet the requirements of IDEA part B.

15. Center for Appropriate Dispute Resolution in Special Education, *IDEA Data Brief: Written State Complaints*, September 2017, https://www.cadreworks.org/sites/default/files/resources/WSC%20Brief_WebFinal_9.2017.pdf.

16. Sally Weale, "Special Needs Pupils in England 'Pushed to One Side' in Covid Crisis," *Guardian*, February 19, 2021, https: //www.theguardian.com/education/2021/feb/19/special-needs-pupils-in-england-pushed-to-one-side-in-covid-crisis.

17. Pooja Pandey and Sumyesh Srivastava, "Excluding the Excluded: India's Response to the Education of Children with Disabilities During Covid-19," *Times of India*, April 26, 2020, https://timesofindia.indiatimes.com/blogs/voices/excluding-the-excluded-indias-response-to-the-education-of-children-with-disabilities-during-covid-19/.

18. Meira Levinson, *Educational Ethics during a Pandemic*, Edmond J. Safra Center for Ethics at Harvard University, May 16, 2020, https://ethics.harvard.edu/files/center-for-ethics/files/17educationalethics2.pdf, 4.

19. Northshore School District, "Letter to Families: Gov. Inslee's Announcement," March 12, 2020, https://www.nsd.org/blog/~board/superintendent-blog/post/letter-to-families-gov-inslees-announcement.

20. John Mooney, "Meeting Remotely, State BOE OKs Remote Learning for Special-Needs Students," *NJ Spotlight News*, April 2, 2020, https://www.njspotlight.com/2020/04/meeting-remotely-state-boe-oks-remote-learning-for-special-needs-students/.

21. Patrick Wall and Devna Bose. "Newark Fails to Enforce Key Special Education Mandates, State Report Says," *Chalkbeat Newark*, November 25, 2019, https://newark.chalkbeat.org/2019/11/25/21109348/newark-fails-to-enforce-key-special-education-mandates-state-report-says.

22. Devna Bose, "As Newark Moves to Virtual Learning, Special Education is an Especially 'Heavy Lift,'" *Chalkbeat Newark*, April 15, 2020, https://newark

.chalkbeat.org/2020/4/15/21225553/as-newark-moves-to-virtual-learning-special-education-is-an-especially-heavy-lift.

23. Natalia Alamdari, "Delaware Public Schools Are Beginning Remote Learning. But Should They Fear Future Lawsuits?" *Delaware Online*, April 1, 2020, https://www.delawareonline.com/story/news/2020/04/01/coronavirus-should-delaware-schools-fear-lawsuits-remote-learning-begins/5094015002/.

24. Erin Richards, "Is Online School Illegal? With Schools Closing from Coronavirus, Special Education Concerns Give Districts Pause," *USA Today*, March 19, 2020, https://www.usatoday.com/story/news/education/2020/03/19/coronavirus-online-school-closing-special-education-teacher-distance-learning/2863503001/.

25. Levinson, *Educational Ethics during a Pandemic*, 6.

26. Richfield Public Schools Distance Learning Comprehensive Guide for Staff, March 18, 2020, obtained via Freedom of Information Act Request. See also Levinson, *Educational Ethics during a Pandemic*, 11.

27. Richards, "Is Online School Illegal?" This concern is not limited to US schools: "Schools in England are using COVID-19 risk assessments as a 'blanket excuse' to prevent pupils with special educational needs and disabilities (SEND) from attending classes." Sally Weale, "English Schools 'Using Coronavirus as Excuse' Not to Teach Special Education Pupils," *Guardian*, July 1, 2020, https://www.theguardian.com/education/2020/jul/01/english-schools-using-coronavirus-as-excuse-not-to-teach-special-needs-pupils. Some other US public school districts rejected online instruction due to equity of access to the needed technology.

28. US Department of Education, "Questions and Answers on Providing Services to Children with Disabilities during the Coronavirus Disease 2019 Outbreak (March 2020)," 2020, https://sites.ed.gov/idea/idea-files/q-and-a-providing-services-to-children-with-disabilities-during-the-coronavirus-disease-2019-outbreak/, answer A-1.

29. US Department of Education, "Supplemental Fact Sheet: Addressing the Risk of COVID-19 in Preschool, Elementary and Secondary Schools While Serving Children with Disabilities," March 21, 2020, https://www2.ed.gov/about/offices/list/ocr/frontpage/faq/rr/policyguidance/Supple%20Fact%20Sheet%203.21.20%20FINAL.pdf, emphasis added.

30. American Association of School Superintendents, "ED Issues Guidance on FAPE During COVID-19," 2020.

31. US Department of Education, Office for Civil Rights, "Fact Sheet: Addressing the Risk of COVID-19 in Schools While Protecting the Civil Rights of Students," March 16, 2020, https://www2.ed.gov/about/offices/list/ocr/docs/ocr-coronavirus-fact-sheet.pdf.

32. US Department of Education, Office for Civil Rights, "Fact Sheet: Addressing the Risk of COVID-19 in Schools While Protecting the Civil Rights of Students."

33. Betsy DeVos, "Recommended Waiver Authority Under Section 3511(d)(4) of Division A of the Coronavirus Aid, Relief, and Economic Security Act ('CARES Act')," US Department of Education, April 27, 2020, https://www2.ed.gov/documents/coronavirus/cares-waiver-report.pdf, 11.

34. See the interactive map here: https://www.edweek.org/leadership/map-coronavirus-and-school-closures-in-2019-2020/2020/03.

35. Executive order 2020–5.

36. Thrun Law Firm P.C. communication to retainer clients including GRPS, obtained via Freedom of Information Act request.

37. E-mail from Laura LaMore to Richard Lemons, May 20, 2020, 4:52 p.m., obtained via Freedom of Information Act request.

38. E-mail from Laura LaMore to SE Admin—LOCAL Supervisors, May 23, 2020, 11:50 a.m., obtained via Freedom of Information Act request.

39. Michigan Governor Executive Order 2020–34.

40. GRPS Implementation Guide: Community of Learning and COVID-19 Response Plan, spring 2020, 3, obtained via Freedom of Information Act request.

41. GRPS Implementation Guide, 3, obtained via Freedom of Information Act request.

42. E-mail from Laura LaMore to Kirsten Myers, May 20, 2020, 10:03 a.m., obtained via Freedom of Information Act request.

43. GRPS, for instance, had 557 students with disabilities whose families did not speak English in the home.

44. Faith Hill, "The Pandemic Is a Crisis for Students with Special Needs," *Atlantic*, April 18, 2020, https://www.theatlantic.com/education/archive/2020/04/special-education-goes-remote-covid-19-pandemic/610231/.

45. Chung, "My Child Has a Disability."

46. US Department of Education, Office of Special Education Programs, "OSEP QA 20–01," September 28, 2020, https://sites.ed.gov/idea/files/qa-provision-of-services-idea-part-b-09-28-2020.pdf, 5.

47. Michigan Governor Executive Order 2020–35, 12. More guidance on compensatory services can be found here: https://sites.ed.gov/idea/idea-files/q-and-a-providing-services-to-children-with-disabilities-during-the-coronavirus-disease-2019-outbreak/.

48. Webb, "Lost Time."

49. Chung, "My Child Has a Disability."

50. Edel Harris, "Lockdown Has Brought Families of Learning Disabled People to Their Knees," *Guardian*, August 11, 2020, https://www.theguardian.com/society/2020/aug/11/lockdown-families-learning-disabled-people-coronavirus.

51. Ami Harbin and Alice MacLachlan, "Pandemic Parenting," *APA Newsletter on Feminism and Philosophy* 20, no. 1 (2020): 23.

52. US Department of Education, Office of Special Education Programs, "OSEP QA 20–01."

53. Kansas State Department of Education, "School Year 2020–21 Compliance with the Individuals with Disabilties Education Act and the Kansas Special Education for Exceptional Children Act for Reopening Schools During the COVID-19 Pandemic," April 1, 2021, https://www.ksde.org/Portals/0/ECSETS/Announcements/COVID-SpEd-FAQ.pdf, 16.

54. Belser, "Disability and the Politics of Vulnerability."

55. *Goldberg v. Kelly*, 397 US. 254 (1970), quoting the preamble to the US Constitution; see also the discussion in Martha Nussbaum, "The Capabilities of People with Cognitive Disabilities," in *Cognitive Diasbility and Its Challenge to Moral Philosophy*, ed. Eva Feder Kittay and Licia Carlson (Malden, MA: Wiley-Blackwell, 2010), 84f.

56. IDEA 1400.c.7.

57. Thanks to Anna Gotlib and Alida Liberman for comments on an earlier version of this chapter.

PART III

Pandemic, Precariousness, and Social Justice

Chapter 7

We Survived COVID-19! (Possibly)

Jamie Lindemann Nelson[1]

This chapter wears a pendant, a short piece that I published late in June of 2020 in the *Hastings Center Report*.[2] As one might expect: short article, ponderous title—"Doubt, Disorientation, and Death in the Plague Time." Yet in my original plan, these words were but a subtitle to the ironically tinged, tabloidesque economy of "I SURVIVED COVID-19 (I Think)"—part of the point of which was to make it plain from the start just whose doubt, disorientation, and death was in question. The wise and compassionate *Report* editors simply ditched the pastiche title and elevated the subtitle to star billing, showing their customary good sense.

This time there is no subtitle.

If I had provided one, though, it would probably have been as turgid (although less alliterative) as my last effort: a list of the present chapter's structural elements (time, derangement, mourning). Old habits die hard. Still, there are differences between the texts. Had the poet T. E. Brown read my first COVID piece, I expect he might have said to me that it was "all replete with very thou"—all about *my* encounter with what was (probably) COVID, *my* struggles with accepting mortality, and concluding with what struck *me* as a consoling insight (if Hamlet's message was, "If it be not now, yet it will come. The readiness is all," mine had more the flavor of, "Ready or not, here it comes"). Something else would need saying about this present piece of writing.

COVID AND EPISTEMIC DERANGEMENT

I'm dwelling on the theme and temperament of the first piece (strongly self-involved, leavened with a splash of wry) to underscore the difference between it and this present writing (socially alert, soberly expressed); making their differences sharper will help me with a sort of diagnostic task that counts as the first order of business here. I take it that there is a widely shared sense that since roughly mid-March of 2020, an enormous shift in our shared life has been compressed into a tiny expanse of time. I hope to unearth an important element of what accounts for that impression.

As it strikes me now, the aims and approach of my first essay, written such a short while ago, seem so utterly overtaken by ensuing events as to now not be merely passé but teetering on the edge of incomprehensibility. That presents a puzzle: What kind of a change could be so calamitous as to sweep an only slightly unruly bit of bioethics to the borders of sense? My suggested resolution carries with it its own challenge: How—and about what—should philosophers write now? The concluding theme on mourning exemplifies a response.

Part of my routine this past year has been to start the day by reading the COVID-related news in the *New York Times*. For the best part of this time, this has been a grim ritual. As the year turned, however, my expectations shifted: There was finally a sensible person at the helm and the virus was meeting its match. Yet it seemed that every positive development was accompanied by something threatening on the other side: New, more transmissible and possibly more deadly versions of the illness were regularly identified; governors of red states pushed to relax restrictions in ways motivated by politics rather than science; the toll of the ill and the dying skyrocketed in India; public health leaders spoke of waiting for the other shoe to drop.

Still, there was a good deal to celebrate. There seemed a sort of magic in the off-the-charts speed with which new, extraordinarily effective and safe vaccines became increasingly available. It was, of course, not sorcery but science that has achieved this astonishing result. Yet so jammed into silos have we become that this great and patent triumph has not decisively allayed the mistrust of upward of 80 million Americans who continue, at the time of this writing, to maintain that they will not be vaccinated (as reported by PBS, NPR, and other news outlets). These refuseniks are thereby contributing to COVID's ability to reinvent itself into new and potentially more lethal varieties, and putting into serious question the chances of achieving herd immunity in this country any time soon.

Many social critics have leveled ethical assaults on vaccine refusal and hesitancy. David Brooks, for example, bewailed the decline of civic virtue it symbolized, the refusal to take the interests of fellow citizens with any seriousness, saying, "We're not asking you to storm the beaches of Iwo Jima; we're asking you to walk into a damn CVS."[3] The use of the expletive by the decorous Brooks conveys exasperation, of course, but the article as a whole makes it plain just what is behind that frustration: Something important about Americans, their willingness to bear burdens for others, something Brooks believes one could count on before, no longer holds.

Yet while I appreciate the significance of ethical critique here, and in particular Brooks's lament about a sea change for the worse in the character of American moral life (none too savory even at its best), my focus here is deeper, or at least different. I am interested in the impact of COVID on the structure of the whole range of concepts that we use to understand and navigate through the world, and of how it stands with us if those concepts cease to be common currency. My chief examples concern what we can know rather than what we ought to do, although the link between the two is deeply important.

What the examples reveal is the depleted state of the reservoirs of trust that support our common life; this includes such major institutions as science and journalism as well as the reasonably good ordering of the many practices and the vast networks of people required to sustain the infusion of such institutions into everyday life. Beyond this there threatens an even deeper defection from basic notions that undergird our ability to go on together, indeed to go on as recognizable selves: consistency, inferential principles, relevance, the bearing of experience on truth, inter alia.

I of course accept that dismantling of accepted norms of rationality is a process that predates the pandemic. Indeed, dissenters from generally accepted views, including views about how views should be assessed, are a commonplace through history—sometimes to humanity's great benefit. Consider, for instance, the shattering views about the character of physical reality that emerged from relativity theory and quantum mechanics in the early part of the twentieth century.

There are traits that, surely, distinguish Albert Einstein's challenge to common sense from that presented by, say, QAnon. But just as surely, it isn't incumbent on anyone to provide a criterion of demarcation that will correctly sort out all the epistemic gold from the dross as a prerequisite for championing relativity and denouncing Q's reprehensible advocacy of a vicious fantasy. Rather, if we were currently in the business of arguing about the matter abstractly, we could say this: Correctly calling the contest between relativity theory and deluded raving would be a test any general account distinguishing reasonable from unreasonable challenges to standing beliefs would need to pass, were it to have any credibility at all.

And then there is the entire social movement that propelled Donald Trump to victory in 2016, that saw him garner close to 75 million votes in defeat in 2020, and that continues to sustain him as a powerful political actor. This movement both enacts and testifies to a yawning chasm in the midst of what has for a long time been a reasonable amount of consensus over which factual claims are true, which false, and what ways of deciding the matter are to be trusted. COVID isn't responsible for all this mess.

Yet even were you to maintain that the sense of rapid and extensive change in our world is primarily attributable to the cultural and political currents that erupted in size of the electorate that voted for Trump—and in the continuing fealty of a major political party to him, despite his shameless lies, his collusion in insurrection, and his manifest unfitness to govern—rather than to COVID, all I'd have to reply would be this: The plague and the president are in relevant respects virtually the same, so tightly have their fates entwined. In Trump's pathetically feckless pandemic response lies much of its success in destroying so many Americans. While Joe Biden's victory may be attributable in no small part to revulsion at Trump's COVID response, consider also the extent to which the innocuous measures to facilitate voting in a pandemic served as a pretext for the Big Lie that holds so many tens of millions in thrall.

In the light of their stunning, blatant success and the potentially mortal stakes of refusal, vaccine denial is in my view an even more portentous indicator that social cohesion is in serious trouble than is the dissensus about the results of the 2020 presidential contest, despite the fact that not a scintilla of supporting evidence has been forthcoming. But if it strikes you the other way round, I'm not going to argue with you. With both of these indicators of cratering trust in play, there is too much else to command our attention.

Yet why might not one's own death—the topic of my earlier paper—count as a reasonable topic for sustained reflection even under such conditions? There doesn't seem to be anything irremediably puzzling or clearly out of order about the enterprise of a person's responding reflectively to the threat of his or her own demise. What kind of a context might be such that it makes thinking so directed so dubious?

Perhaps one in which there are credible and pressing existential threats to something whose significance dwarfs an individual's death. Vaccine denial threatens the lives of hundreds of thousands. Yet if this insensitivity to the social is the sort of thing that can make an otherwise reasonably well-behaved bioethics article seem a senseless performance, then the literature of the field is simply stuffed with senselessness.

I think the nature of the threat confronting us in COVID's wake is graver than even the loss of many lives; in danger are the structures providing us all with the necessary conditions for living lives about which it makes sense to care, to strive to save and to preserve, to mourn for and to hold in memory.

These structures include norms of belief formation and of valuation, norms of recollection and of hope. Shared norms of these kinds make it possible for societies to discern opportunities and threats and to make and assess strategies of response, allowing individuals to dispute those discernments and challenge the strategies. They make possible art and play, reflection and relaxation, passion and repose. In the absence of significant degrees of consensus on many of these norms, social life and very likely our individual lives as psychological subjects are in peril.

In his discussion of the grounds of what humans can be sure of, Wittgenstein speaks of "agreement not in opinions but in form of life."[4] Among many ideas suggested by this gravid piece of prose is the notion that the agreements that support all our knowledge and that give point to all our doubts are not typically subject to the give and take of life's ordinary disputations, that they are part of the structure of what it is to be a human being. They include such things as the confidence that the future will resemble the past in ways that we can recognize, that human beings in general have rich interior lives, that in addition and other forms of inferential thinking, we are guided by a certain common understanding of what is relevant that excludes strange conclusions that logic alone arguably permits. Of the many ways in which the current sense that "we" (in the Global North, in the United States) have "beaten" COVID could turn out to have been overstated, premature, or simply wrong, what seems to me most worrisome is how the pandemic has exposed deep fissures in our form of life, and in exposing them has driven them yet deeper.

So much for why the first COVID piece seems now to be just so altogether beside the point: Its individualism leaves no room for grappling with our "real need." Yet this leaves us with another question, particularly pointed for those who have devoted much of their lives to the task of writing essays of that rough sort. If, indeed, we face a threat to our hopes of going on together in a way that affords us the opportunity to make sense of the world and to the world, of ourselves and to ourselves, what, if anything, should now be the aim of essays in philosophy—and in particular, in socially engaged philosophy?

I think there are fine answers to analogous questions for artists; their work seeks to introduce into the world objects that people will think worthy of attending to, often of admiring, even loving, quite for the sake of the objects themselves. Additionally, the work of artists and their interpreters can provide rich occasions for understanding others better even when we don't share their enthusiasm for a particular instance or form of artistic expression—and when what delights and inspires us leaves them cold. All this work seems on the side of the angels, providing a potentially unifying counter to the widening gyre, implicitly reminding us of what we share, as well as replenishing the store of items we may appreciate together.

Something along similar lines might be said of other disciplines that aim to uncover, clarify, and systematically display truths about the world. Every feature of reality that we can more confidently acknowledge and set more firmly into a shareable worldview may contribute to the security with which people accept common terms of reference. They might also be useful dialectically, at least for those whose skepticism of the real and infatuation with the fantastic has not gone so far as to render them invulnerable to the sting in the tail of cognitive dissonance.

But what of philosophy, a practice not celebrated for its ability to engender consensus, but one that prides itself on its tendency to follow the argument wherever it may lead? Do we really want professionals highly skilled at devising ingenious ways of subjecting our conceptual structures to destructive stress tests, to go about their business as usual, when they notoriously are much less able to generate agreement that the concepts in question—significant notions such as truth, reality, value, death, gender, knowledge, freedom—are in good repair?

One good reason for saying yes is traceable at least back to David Hume, who argued in his *Enquiry concerning Human Understanding* that the work of philosophers typically passes by in obscurity, undetected by the vast majority of people. Another, perhaps better reason is that no one has legitimate authority to issue any cease-and-desist orders to philosophers, nor would any effort to do so likely be effective, if history is any guide.

It's open to philosophers to say that their work draws on and reinforces standards of rationality every bit as much as work by physicists, and any burden of explaining the paucity of received results achieved by philosophers contrasted to scientists is shared with sociologists, literary critics, economists, and many other kinds of academic workers—so there! Yet one might hope for a less defensive reply.

Is there an epistemology of anger and disaffection that might help us better understand how belief and evidence can become so estranged? Are there distinctive forms of value, or circumstances in which evaluation is called for, when shared frameworks are unavailable in which philosophical reflection might be of help? Are there special challenges to acting well in the wake of the pandemic that are hard to see? What answer might we now make to Immanuel Kant's third great question: What may we hope for? What answer to its silent shadow? What should we dread?

In the remainder of this chapter, I want to take up the question of how to understand mourning, specifically concerning the losses that we've suffered jointly as a result of the trail COVID cut among us and of the even greater loss it might occasion. I want to point to some disturbing features of mourning that, again, can't all be laid at COVID's door, but which may be made vivid in its light. And I want to suggest ways in which mourning, like art, might possibly serve as a counterweight to the forces that are degrading our common life. Our real needs are numerous and weighty, but not easy to specify or to rank. Along the way I hope to make a case why getting clearer about how we ought to respond to grave loss is a part of what we really need now.

MOURNING, GRIEVING, AND COVID

Some preliminaries: it's typically claimed that grief is an emotion triggered by irredeemable loss of something greatly valued, while mourning is the expression of grief in terms that are socially recognizable and even ritualized. I don't want to deny this. Yet it seems possible to be a mourner who is not a griever, without one's mourning being a piece of hypocrisy. One might feel mournful about something, might mourn the passing of someone, in a fashion that acknowledges the irremediable loss of something of unique and irreplaceable value without thereby grieving it.

Or so I claim. Recall the last time you attended a sporting event and were asked to observe a moment of silence for the latest victim of police violence or fallen first responder, or to say her name, to rescue from obscurity another woman of color killed by racist misogyny. You were invited to participate in a shared ritual of mourning. But is your voluntary participation necessarily an expression of grief?

This is not at all to deny the vividness of your experience, the sincerity of your revulsion about the little value dominant strains of American culture place on Black lives, your sympathy for the firefighter who died by fire, the wholeheartedness of your mourning. Rather it is to draw attention to different features of the concepts. Consider their relationship to time. One can mourn for a moment—a moment of silence—but grief is not so punctual a condition. The notion of being seized with grief for a precise, clockable, brief moment seems to miss something crucial about grief and its place in our lives.

Two thoughts might seem to explain this difference:

1. Mourning is the social expression of any appropriate affective or cognitive response to grave and irrecoverable loss that befalls us or those with whom we identify. As a basically communicative act, mourning's relationship to time is easily understood.
2. Mourning has a social dimension, to be sure, but it also is a component of our inner lives: A person could be said to be mourning the loss of a loved one compatible with a vast range of actions and inactions, none of which need involve what you wear or standing in solidarity with others, or bearing any palls at all. In fact, with regard to this inner dimension

> we might be inclined to say that grief and mourning are distinguished only by the intensity of the associated affect.

As it happens, I cordially dislike both these accounts. I think it does scant justice to the lived reality of either grief or mourning to assign one exclusively to an elusive private realm, while the other is altogether public. If you're in search of a counterexample in the form of a piece of behavior that clearly and distinctly counts as grieving and not mourning, I think the best I might do is to remind you of how natural it might be to speak of the violence of a person's grief. "Violent mourning," on the other hand, puts one in mind of what some unusual color of nail polish might be labeled, or of a Monty Pythonesque spat during a graveside service.

The proposal that the two concepts can be distinguished in terms of the intensity of feelings fares no better. Consider the situation of a person whose grief has left them "hollowed out," so to speak, and insensible to any distinctive, vivid feeling. I think it may be said of both grief and mourning what is more commonly said of anger: They are each compatible with very many feelings—and even with none at all.

In my own view, it makes more sense to chart out the relationship between these notions by getting clearer about what I earlier referred to as their place in our lives. What do we need distinguishable concepts of grief and mourning to do for us? And how might either or both notions help us mend the cracks that threaten to shatter our form of life?

I start with an observation about how the yawning epistemic gaps between people in the United States are not randomly distributed but have a tight correlation with certain demographic markers, such as class, education, race, residence, and, most powerfully, political affiliation. Insofar as folks are aware of these gaps, there is a tendency to see them as reflecting roughly the image that I have Jeremiaded about throughout. People stare across a widening distance at each other, on both sides with the feeling that only some fundamental difference between them could explain such a massive disagreement. I fear this as much as anything right now: that the conceptual disagreement among us will drive a sense that we do not share a single form of life—a thought that has a tragic legacy.

What might either grief or mourning do for us not merely as responses appropriate to marking the crumbling of essential features we share in common, but as reasonable efforts to lessen or even to stop those sands from further shifting? Consider my urging artistic expression as a worthy object of pursuit, even in times that wear an apocalyptic tinge, on the grounds that in trying to create states, events, objects, or processes that are valuable for their own sake, they might just replenish the stock of what we care about while reminding us that even if we don't value the same things, the very ability to value things in this noninstrumental fashion represents a distinctive recurring theme in this form of life. Both replenishment and reminder might exert centripetal force against the winds threatening to blow us apart.

If anyone noticed in response to this that among the aspirations animating many leading contemporary artists, knitting an on-the-ropes culture back together isn't conspicuous, it was kind of you not to make a fuss, but to read on. Notwithstanding, I want to make a similar argument on behalf of our need to mark loss, so rather than enter the cudgels directly on behalf of art, I'll concentrate on the grievous and the mournful.

In a powerful article in *Philosophy and Public Affairs*, Dan Moller notes a feature of grief not often remarked on, at least within moral psychology: We tend to get over it quickly—perhaps even more quickly than we ought. As Moller notes, a striking percentage of bereaved husbands and wives find themselves in new and satisfying intimate relationships a year after the death of their former spouses.[5]

Moller seems to be of the opinion that there is something disturbing in the apparent readiness of people to move on so rapidly from the loss of someone with whom they had been committed to share their entire lives. I feel much the same, although I'm less clear than he seems to be about just what disturbs me here.

One possibility is that I simply find it indecorous, that it offends my sensibilities about what's fitting. Another is that it violates a moral norm in that it is a failure to live so as to vindicate the understandings implicit in professions of love. (Wittgenstein again is apt here: "Love is not a feeling. Love is put to the test, pain, not. One does not say: 'That was not true pain, or else it would not have gone off so quickly.'")[6] The strength and persistence of my grief is, on this account, love's last great test.

I find this a telling insight, and am nudged by it to see both grief and mourning as human practices that are directly morally assessable, by which I mean that each enterprise is open to question concerning the propriety of its exercise, its proper objects, its coherence with other attitudes, and so forth. ("Indirectly morally assessable," as I use the notions, would go to such matters as whether and to what extent the fact that one was mourning or grief-stricken might serve to excuse or mitigate otherwise blameworthy actions.)

While I am of a mind to think that a person's mourning or grief can be assessed in ethical terms, I also find it much easier to think about such cases in aretaic rather than deontic modes—which is to say that norms concerning who, what, when, why, and how we are to mourn or grieve are grounded in the actions, thoughts, and emotions of virtuous people rather than codified in lists of principles. (Consider how many clauses specifying exceptions, qualifications, and conditions there would have to be!)

We all are subject to the kind of losses that are open to grief and mourning. We all therefore face challenges as to who and how and why we grieve and mourn. Insofar as we accept that an aretaic way of thinking holds the key to how such challenges are to be answered, we will be on the lookout for the grieving *sophron*, the mourning *phronimos*, the bereaved person of practical wisdom to help us meet the challenges well.

There is, I hasten to add, nothing easy about this, no reason for thinking that vivid reminders of how the significance and sense of our lives are bound up with the lives of others will surely renew and expand our sense that, when it all comes down to dust, we are all in this together, that what we share is more important than what rives us. For now, even grief has become political, and what one mourns is a function of what one values.

Yet suppose we consider just the 720,000 lives lost in the United States alone and think about those people and their deaths for a moment, wondering how should we respond to a tragedy of this magnitude. Since 1775–246 years—the United States has lost in the neighborhood of 670,000 lives to combat. COVID has cost us more than that in less than a year and a half. How should we grieve this glut of death; how ought we, collectively, begin to mourn these people? And as we are thinking here of these modes of bereavement as open to moral assessment, we might be inclined to think of the invitation at the start of this paragraph as far from innocent: COVID has killed roughly 4 million of us worldwide. What gives us the right to distinguish among all the dead 15 percent who merit deeper mourning, graver grief?

It is true that COVID is so contentious a disease that we might be thought to be doing well to undergo any bereavement at all for any of its victims. Yet the experience of grief and the impulse to mourn are such strong and pervasive features of our form of life that encountering them in others' lives should serve to renew the sense of what is common in human experience. Making this vivid and tracing out its implications could well be a fitting task for philosophers in this harsh time, as well as for artists and critics, historians and classicists, scholars of religion and of the human sciences.

There are no guarantees, of course. One of the powerful contrasts between the forty-fourth and forty-fifth presidents is precisely in their mourning of deaths that had a public character to them. Contrast Barack Obama's response to the slayings at Mother Emanuel church with the reports of Trump's seemingly sincere puzzlement over the death of US soldiers in the nation's wars: What could those suckers possibly have been motivated by, what was in it for them? If that man is the *phronimos* of the vaccine deniers, if it is his overwhelming narcissism that is their guiding star, then perhaps even the most emotionally subtle and intellectually sound effort to remind us of the importance of the fact that we all are moved by the deaths of at least someone may end up making us more lonely.

And if all I could well hope for comes from the keyboards of philosophers and playwrights, from artists' studios and archeologist's digs, that would not necessarily get us farther in the struggle for notions of a sound human understanding lodged in human lives soundly lived. Should everyone awake from this bad dream tomorrow, that would not usher in a ceremony of innocence. What we look for now is only a therapy against a specific disease, not a panacea.

Perhaps even less: perhaps all we can get is a heightened sense of how precarious our situation is, of the range of threats to our survival of COVID-19, of how uncertain of their aims are the strategies I've roughed out. I can easily imagine even a well-intentioned reader wondering here if I haven't been too alarmist in my reading of the consequences of even fundamental forms of disagreement, and if not, too naive in thinking that any of the responses I sketched have a chance in hell of working.

To the first, all I have to say is, let it be so! To the second, a bit more. The target of these remarks includes, perhaps quixotically, the hard-core Trumpists, QAnon fanciers, and vaccine denialists. However, the chief target is the "woke"—people who like me think that all those folks are wrong, wrong, foolishly, dangerously, reprehensibly wrong. That they are so is clear. But whether we should toss them all into a basket of deplorables is something that, however tempting, I warn against. People do and say and believe deplorable things, surely: deplorable both because their actions and pronouncements and beliefs are bigoted or otherwise open to the strongest ethical condemnation, and because there is virtually nothing that plausibly can be urged on their behalf. But to think of the authors of those sayings and the doers of those deeds as themselves deplorable is to take another step, particularly if in taking that step we simultaneously are covertly congratulating ourselves on just how delightfully nondeplorable we happen to be. This is not a case against ever holding people accountable for their choices—just a gentle plea not to let thoughts grow in us that make it more difficult to see that despite the seemingly enormous distances between us, the gaps are all human sized. If we can hang on to that thought, we may be able to say that we as a form of life did just barely manage to survive COVID-19.

NOTES

1. Without the assistance of Eric Nelson, I should not have been able to write this paper; I'm also indebted to Hilde Lindemann for her suggestions after the reading of an early draft.

2. Jamie Lindemann Nelson, "Doubt, Disorientation, and Death in the Plague Time," *Hastings Center Report* 50, no. 3 (May/June 2020): 4.

3. David Brooks, "Our Herd Immunity Failure," *New York Times*, May 7, 2021.
4. Wittgenstein, Ludwig, and G E. M. Anscombe. *Philosophical Investigations*. (Oxford, UK: Blackwell, 1997).
5. Dan Moller, "Wealth, Disability and Happiness," *Philosophy and Public Affairs* 39, no. 2 (spring 2011): 177–206.
6. Ludwig Wittgenstein, *Zettel*, trans. G. E. M. Anscombe, eds. G. E. M. Anscombe and G. H. von Wright (Oxford: Blackwell, 1967), §504.

Chapter 8

New Labors, New Burdens: Care Work Re-narrated

Jennifer Scuro

I suggest that illness is not only a life event that can be studied by philosophy, but also a forceful invitation to philosophise.

—Havi Carel[1]

Disability is a reservoir of knowledge.

—David Mitchell, Sharon Snyder and Linda Ware[2]

I DON'T WANT A "NEW NORMAL" OR TO GO "BACK TO NORMAL"

I've become quite suspicious of anyone who invests energy and resources in wanting a "return to normal," or whose desires for normalcy have become a way to think through or about this pandemic.[3] If we account for it honestly, 2020 was a year that marked the beginning of an event of mass death.[4] There were social and political preconditions operative (ones that were, for me, particularly personal and professional) before the onset of the global pandemic, making the suspension of normalcy easily perceived as permissible, as a moral obligation. We had to stop everything—especially those of us who were primarily responsible for the care of others. Those of us laboring already in ways that follow an alternative narrative about what it means to care, to be tasked as the one that someone else depends upon for their day-to-day survival, were "accustomed" to these kinds of interruptions—no matter how uncomfortable—and would have to hack the system in our day-to-day labors in ways quite different from the norm. Simply stated, the pace and expectations of everyday life were arrested for everyone else because of the pandemic, but I had already been experiencing it years before—and with increasing acuity.

In 2019, the institution that employed me closed down, and a more-than-twenty-year-long career came to a grinding halt. Along with all the other responsibilities of being a wife and mother, I was the primary caretaker of a nonneurotypical child in crisis. I already had an extended network of family and friends with whom I found strong bonds of mutual aid. Being unemployed added to the depth of the stress and despair of not feeling that I could do enough to keep everyone well and safe. While trying to perform a kind of "pleasant productivity"[5] and the *appearance* of wellness, my mental health declined, effects of PTSD took a toll on my body and metabolism, and my ability to rest had eroded.

My spouse, a bus operator—now considered a "frontline worker"—was also made aware of the radical precarity of the situation without much room for agency as he regularly drove past the refrigerator trucks full of dead bodies outside of NewYork Presbyterian Queens Hospital in Flushing, New York. What he witnessed—and what many who were considered on the front lines of the pandemic also witnessed—was the helplessness even of those in the best position to help.

This pervasive feeling of helplessness, combined with despair of having nothing (or at least very little) to look forward to, are the two prongs of concern that I hope to address here. Specifically, I focus on (1) the way in which helplessness is both a suffering and a political construction of white saviorism, now magnified by the pandemic, and (2) the complicated labor that comes with thinking about and planning for the future when one is disabled in the context of a society that thinks, more often than not, that "it is better to be dead than disabled."[6]

As the pandemic unfolded in New York, in what was one of the first "epicenters" of the pandemic in the United States,[7] I witnessed others around me, as well as on social media, express a similar twofold despair. This frustrated me because it meant there were now political teeth in the idea that there is value only in being "useful" and "helpful." That is, in a culture already dangerously ableist and somatophobic,[8] to be unemployed or underemployed can be a source of shame and despair;[9] to be unemployed and disabled can be life-threatening in the sense that there is pervasive assumption that there is "no future"[10] for those who cannot conform or appear to be able-bodied. As Robert McRuer terms it, in "Compulsory Able-Bodiedness and Queer/Disabled Existence,"

> Like compulsory heterosexuality, . . . compulsory able-bodiedness functions by covering over, with the appearance of choice, a system in which there actually is no choice. . . . [A] system of compulsory able-bodiedness . . . emanates from everywhere and nowhere. . . .
>
> [Able]-bodied culture . . . assumes in advance that we all agree: able-bodied identities, able-bodied perspectives are preferable and what we all, collectively, are aiming for. A system of compulsory able-bodiedness repeatedly demands that people with disabilities embody for others an affirmative answer to the unspoken question. Yes, but in the end, wouldn't you rather be more like me?[11]

In resistance to this, it is important to suss out what McRuer terms here "compulsory able-bodiedness" as an operative, implicit, and invisible set of assumptions about normality in our social and political frameworks, now rendered stranger and more arbitrary in pandemic conditions.

There is an abundance of literature and testimony as to why and how we could renarrate these perceptions of able-bodiedness, free of the existential threats to remain productive at all costs. More than that, I would like to claim that, especially after this first year of a global pandemic, we *ought to take instruction* from those who already know how to "crip" the system[12]—a strategy that reclaims and subverts those demands for normality away from compulsory able-bodiedness as well as from the branding and whitewashing of "health and well-being" common to these pervasive ableist cultural perceptions. In this way, following Critical Disability Studies scholarship and the methodology of "cripping," I suggest that it is essential to "flip the script" so that we neither need nor want to "return to normal," nor ought we spend precious labor seeking out how to configure a "new normal" as a path to some neoliberal phantasm of "recovery."[13]

To be disabled means that so much of the everyday is already "unsurvivable." Philosopher Helen De Cruz[14] cites blind fiction writer Robert Kingett because he raises some important concerns about the return to normal in relation to his work community. His concerns and observations seem quite fair. From Kingett:

> I can't stop thinking about how the world will go back to normal once the virus goes away. When the world goes back to the way it was, this will give [my] industry even more chances to be the gatekeepers they've always wanted to become. . . .
>
> I hope things stay as they are—remote, and accessible to all regardless of geographic location. I'm dreading the day non-disabled people will go back to their normal lives because that will leave me, and so many like me, shut out to a greater degree than before. . . .

> Sure, we still have a long way to go, but the pandemic has proven that our system is deeply broken and can in fact change to make lives easier with very minimal effort.[15]

Turning to Crip Theory within the Critical Disability Studies scholarship, there is an important, underrepresented historical narrative about the maintenance of normalcy "at all costs." It is harmful, grief-inducing, and unsustainable. To become a "burden" or to be perceived as part of a larger "free rider" problem is met with considerable viciousness, including anger, fear, and disgust, complicated by those additional layers of internalized ableism. This narrative manifests grief-inducing harms with traumatic effect, holding the weight of the harmful assumptions given to anyone not considered "productive" and "hardworking," but rather, as if their being-in-the-world is only "burdensome" and "tragic."

When it comes to care labor—the invisible emotional and intellectual labors of survival in particular—that deals with and resists these ableist ideas of unevenly distributed "burdensomeness," disabled people have already been doing this work. It is labor that already shares in the same old dangerous and deadly intersections of anti-Black racism, heteronormativity, queerantagonism, and the like. There is a creative power of resistance that opens up liminal spaces, even when systems fail, emerging from this intense labor. We assume the burden of failure is on the individual and neglect the urgency and need to change the system when individuals cannot maintain these normative expectations. Yet, as Cyborg-poet Jillian Weise describes it, "as a cyborg, I think about space in a really liberatory way. I think about digital space. . . . I think about hacks, how to get in sideways, and in that sense it's exciting."[16]

What follows are my musings and tentative responses to questions that have come from the twofold problem I had been thinking about prepandemic, now amplified. This is also my way to hack through the grief of becoming burdensome, compensating for my perceived "loss of value." I do not respond to these questions in a comprehensive way here at all; rather, these are "tinkerings"[17] with the explicit intention of engaging in antiableist challenges to a political economy that shapes our lifeworld in terms of market value expectations underwritten with the assumed entitlements for those who embody neoliberal ideals. I found myself more and more often asking:

- Who is most burdened by invisible labor?
- How are these labors distributed?
- Can we or should we try to "escape" from the burdens of invisible labors?
- How do we value work in a time of crisis?

- How have some lives become less grievable and more precarious? Or, more importantly, how has the pandemic made our (paid and unpaid) work more precarious and easier to exploit?[18]

In short, my responses to these questions of labor—its distributions, its implicit ableism, the desire to escape in the context of being disabled and unemployed during the pandemic-as-crisis—so far are quite partial. I start at the point of this new quality of helplessness, accessing these questions by first renarrating what it means to be both helpful and helpless. Because the current crisis is also a crisis in care and care labor, I think it becomes important to "hack" our understanding of time, akin to Weise's hacking of space, especially because the everyday pace of things, in the midst of a pandemic, seems to have failed. That the temporality of our work may be irrevocably changed and may not be recovered in the same way again, from a disabled perspective, can be quite liberating. It is important to reconcile the suspension of these everyday perceptions of being-in-the-world made available by the pandemic, because these perceptions and desires remain dangerously ableist. I think this danger is evidenced by this persistent but ultimately questionable desire to return to normal.

HELPLESSNESS IS A KIND OF SUFFERING (AND A POLITICAL CONSTRUCTION)

This past year demonstrated a crisis in care: in how we care for those who precariously labor, in how the burdens of care labor are distributed, and in what is valuable in the sustainment and outcomes of these labors. Interpreted by an ableist, neoliberal culture—which protects a violent individualism in which it is best when one "needs no help"—we began to mythologize "heroes out of helpers." It is a mythology that is closely tied to the idea of American exceptionalism.[19] It is also one that is hard to counter with a critical perspective, and provides "apolitical" cover for those with the most political power and socioeconomic benefit while further burdening those who are most precarious and disabled. This veil of benevolence was pulled the moment Jeff Bezos, upon his return from a brief space flight in the middle of a global pandemic, stated, "I want to thank every Amazon employee and every Amazon customer, 'cause you guys paid for all this." This, with full knowledge of Amazon's notorious history of labor violations,[20] deflects the responsibility for the real risks which its "essential workers" have unnecessarily lived with since March 2020.

In an ableist neoliberal society, in which labor is valued in terms of capital and expendable labor, all efforts are valued in the direction of their market benefits. As a consequence, it is assumed to be a moral good when one is in a position to help, whether in the ordinary course of business or in the extraordinary conditions of crisis. As Mister Rogers was known for telling young children when they were exposed to crisis, "Look for the helpers. You will always find people helping."[21]

The "one who helps" is understood to be in a position of benign independence, freely able to move between interest, choice, and charity—an entitlement of discretionary care. In a position to help, I can choose how much to care, but also can choose when to withdraw care. I can be arbitrary and self-affirmed in my position as helping and, ironically, even if I harm, I can absolve myself if my intention was "pure," because I "just wanted to help." Conversely, if one needs help, or merely is not in a position to help—or is simply not "able"—this can render one suspicious and even blameworthy.

We have come to view that to be in a position to help, and to want to labor in service to others,[22] is a most rewardable position. In the early days of the pandemic, there were daily calls to show appreciation for health care workers worldwide—7:00 p.m. nightly became the designated New York City time. There was also a unique phenomenon that accompanied the work of "first responders" and "hero" helpers, as described by Ross K. Baker for *USA Today*:

> What must be the cruelest and most confounding thing about death in this pandemic is the inability of family and friends to gather close to the bedside of a dying loved one. Viewing the family member or friend separated by a double-pane window in an intensive care unit, or from outside the building, or by closed-circuit television, would be the very denial of the "good death," were it not for the overburdened and exhausted nurses and doctors swaddled in protective clothing.[23]

Yet the testimonies on social media of healthcare workers as the virus-ravaged cities and communities became a source of an important insight: those who were trained, prepared, and in the best position to help were rendered tragically helpless (see figure 1), inducing a unique labor of trauma and grief attached to this difficult work.[24] I suggest that this kind of helplessness, without sustained and established care communities of mutual aid, becomes a novel form of unnecessary and useless suffering.[25]

Consider the waged or newly designated "frontline" workers. For them, there was a new mode of alienation, shaping a novel mode of worker exploitation that opened up opportunities for real victimization. Take, for example, the case of Jason Hargrove, a Detroit bus driver who took to social media in March 2020 to call out a coughing rider. Only a few weeks later, Hargrove died of COVID-19 (see figure 2). The position of the first-responder-as-hero

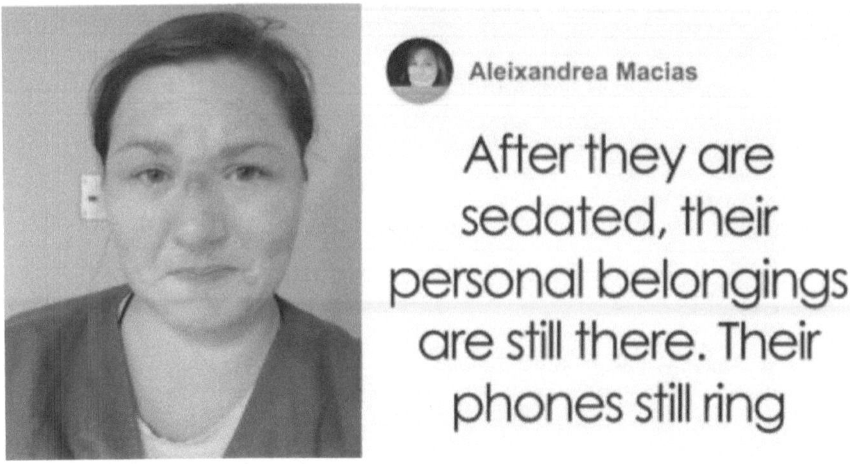

Figure 8.1 Aleixandrea Macias sharing her experience of working in an ICU, pictured on social media: a white woman, crying, with marks on her nose from her PPE, wearing blue scrubs next to the black-and-white text of her testimony stating, "After they are sedated, their personal belongings are still there. Their phones still ring." ***Aleixandrea Macias's Facebook post***

constructed a false narrative of obligation to care at the risk of many a marginalized worker not granted the means for advocacy or self-care and protection from the harms of exposure to greater precarities than are conscionable.

Despite any possible good intentions, a binary emerges which implies that with the praise we give to dedicated helpers comes a kind of perceived "moral failing" of those who "do not help"—whether one interferes with help, cannot help, needs help, refuses help, or even if one finds oneself helpless. This binary between the helper and those that need help, magnified by the pandemic, for me, raises a question: Isn't there a serious error in the way we build tropes around this binary?

This binarization embedded in the dynamics of care, organized by who is helpful and who is helpless, I would argue, leads to the misperception and ableist attitudes about the constitution of care labors, especially because it is often assumed that the need for help can begrudgingly beget burdensomeness and unnecessary labors. Disability justice advocate and writer Rachel Cohen-Rottenberg already had warned that disabled people were always in danger of being turned into "help objects,"[26] made vulnerable to caretakers and aid workers who are waged to "help" the "helpless." The history of this binary between those "who help" and those "who need help" is rife with racism, ableism, paternalism, and eugenic ideologies.[27] This error in thinking is as harmful as it is indiscriminate, whether one is perceived as "helpless" or just simply as someone who "cannot help themselves."[28] It results in the

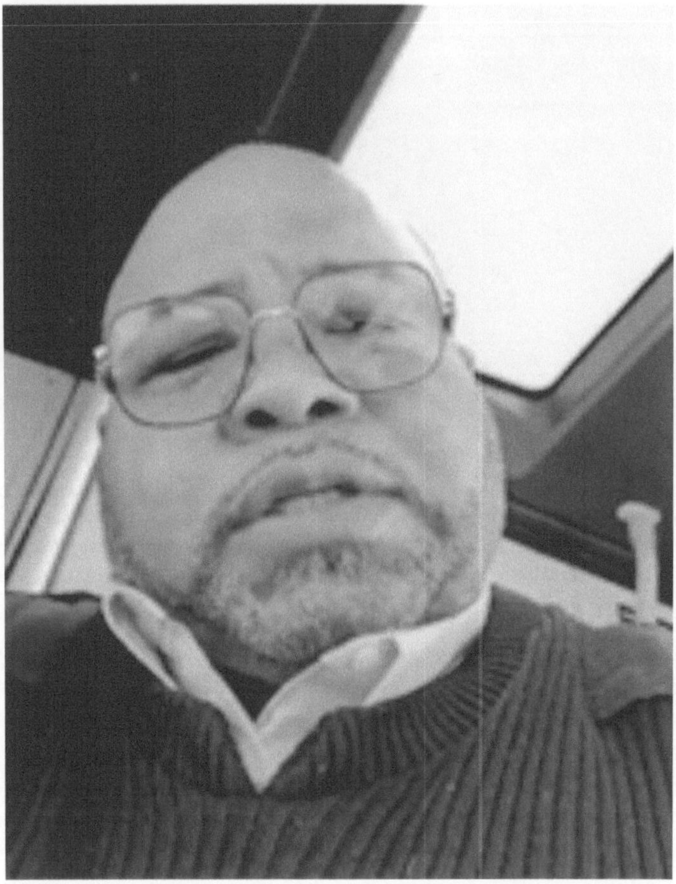

Figure 8.2 A screengrab of Jason Hargrove, a Black man in a bus operator uniform and glasses, speaking into the camera on social media. ***Courtesy of Desha Hargrove***

reluctance to help others with the preference to only "help oneself," regardless of who might be most in need.

Following McRuer and Johnson, I would like to suggest that we resource an important critique of neoliberalism offered by Critical Disability Studies, specifically as the critique comes out of the framework of Crip Theory:

> The shifting economy under neoliberalism is . . . about service and exhausting affective labor (smile! take care of me!)—labor that continues to be gendered female. Crip theory in this crisis should ask who cares: literally, who performs service work, but also, more coarsely, who gives a shit about you and your need to be smiled at? Which bodies/minds/impairments in this moment of crisis will count as authentically and publicly disabled? Which will not? How will disability and impairment be measured? Thinking about all of this in the twenty-first

> century requires attending to many topics of [conversation:] . . . movements in search of theories; mad turns; illegible disabilities; dysregulated emotions; the state's power to produce, contain, deny, or (mis)recognize impairment; disability beyond or across borders.[29]

If the maximum intended effect of helping is to "do no harm," then to help in a meaningful way is a practice of judgment that includes knowledge, experience, and habituation. Effective helping practices require an openness to constant correction in a context of mutual aid—this is labor that is expensive but ought not make us expendable; it is a potential creative and renewable resource against some of the most exhausting of care labors; it is the work that is horrendously undervalued in a society that has privatized and monetized all care relations.

Theorist Silvia Federici already understood—prepandemic—the ways in which "everyday life" can be a state of "permanent crisis" and that, in the context of care work, everyday life "has been allowed to shipwreck."[30] She argues that "to de-politicize labor" is to allow it to go "unwaged," suggesting instead that we need to "reconstruct the commons" and engage in "anti-privatization" campaigns. Federici also argues that "[a]s the capitalist crisis destroys the basic elements of reproduction for millions of people across the world, including the United States, the reconstruction of our everyday life is a possibility and a necessity."[31]

This was the first and most provocative prompt for me to reconsider the burdens of privatized, everyday care labors beyond the dynamic of the helpless/helpful binary, especially in the wake of a pandemic. As the *New York Times* describes it, Federici already had explained in the 1970s that our reproductive labors provide a site for exploitation.[32] She argued in "Wages against Housework" (1975) that there is an "emotional tax" in the way gender roles are naturalized through unwaged work, performed "in the name of love" and out of care, so much so that "our bodies and emotions are distorted for [this] special function."[33]

Case in point, as described in a statement by UNWomen.org:

> Women who are poor and marginalized face an even higher risk of COVID-19 transmission and fatalities, loss of livelihood, and increased violence. Globally, 70 per cent of health workers and first responders are women, and yet, they are not at par with their male counterparts. At 28 per cent, the gender pay gap in the health sector is higher than the overall gender pay gap (16 per cent).[34]

This kind of unwaged care labor and service work still does not carry the right of refusal: "jobs women perform are mere extensions of the housewife's condition . . . we become nurses, maids, teachers, secretaries . . . [and] the fact that people's lives depend on us, [it becomes impossible] to see where our work begins and ends, where our work ends and our desires begin."[35] To this I add: the economic risks beget existential risks and the kinds of everyday labors needed—because they are often without the right of refusal—require renegotiation because they are dangerous in their *burdensomeness*, enforcing and sustaining economic, political, and existential precarities for some but not distributed evenly to all.[36]

Fast-forward from 1975 to 2008, Federici shifts focus to the way these burdensome labors amplify risk and precarity: "The triumph of neoliberalism has worsened this situation . . . [by] destroying subsistence economies and making millions dependent on monetary incomes."[37] The dominant expectation is that these labors continue to go unwaged, unchallenged, as they drain and exhaust those who are expected to perform them. This is evident from the studies of the disadvantaging of women in the pandemic not only in terms of their economic and career prospects but also in existential terms as embodied beings for whom health risks are great—even greater for women of color and working-class women—and for whom quality of life is directly related to our survival.[38]

PANDEMIC TIME IS ALSO "CRIP TIME"[39]

The scholarship of Critical Disability Studies has so much to offer in the way we can imagine what comes next, postpandemic. Queer disabled writer, performance artist, and advocate Leah Lakshmi Piepzna-Samarasinha describes this in their book *Care Work: Dreaming Disability Justice* by naming a "crip emotional intelligence" to capture how valuable the labor was in the hacks of surviving everyday ableist expectations:

> [All] the crip skills I was seeing and learning that I and other disabled folks had . . . meant something because, well, the deficiency model by which most people view disability only sees disabled people as a lack, a defect, damaged good, in need of a cure. The idea that we have cultures, skills, science, and technology runs counter to all that. In a big way.[40]

There is a special kind of knowledge that comes from crip survivorship, as well as the joyful ways to create and sustain collective care. This includes the narratives of "crip time" and the many facets of crip emotional intelligence, as Piepzna-Samarasinha describes it. In the wake of the pandemic, one of those facets stands out for me:

> Crip emotional intelligence is understanding isolation. Deeply. We know what it's like to be really, really alone. To be forgotten about, in that way where people just don't remember you've ever been out, at meetings and parties, in the social life of the world. How being isolated, being shunned, being cut off from the social world of community is terrifying because you know that it can literally kill you. And that being alone also does not always have to be killing; it can also be an oasis of calm, quiet, low stimulation, and rest.[41]

A special feature of this politically constructed suffering of helplessness that adds to the crisis of a pandemic is *isolation*—isolation from community and isolation from ease of access to sources of mutual aid. It is what I have termed elsewhere, a "phenomenon of dismemberment,"[42] and for me signals a more suspicious problem: that the dangerous and deadly invisible mechanisms of ableism are latent yet operative, amplified by the fact that, as Federici puts it, "capitalism fosters a permanent reproduction crisis."[43] The care and service labor that sustains the bodies and minds of those most vulnerable, instead of being understood as a potentially renewable resource, is fully devalued in the wake of privatized interests and market demands.

At the heart of the instruction that I suggest we take from Crip Theory, in taking the opportunity to resist the new reproductive crises of a global pandemic, is the idea of "crip time." Disability scholar Ellen Samuels outlines an excellent account of crip time as the radically different pace and texture of time that comes out of disabled living, a way of resisting an economic and social fabric that expects—or rather, prizes—individualized independence and able-bodiedness. Citing Alison Kafer, Samuels recounts that "rather than bend disabled bodies and minds to meet the clock, crip time bends the clock to meet disabled bodies and minds."[44]

One facet of her "six ways of looking at" crip time includes her claim that "crip time is writing time."[45] Within the context of what I am calling a "crip survivorship," there is a valid and biting critique of neoliberalism, in which much of the labor of resistance is already done and in which one can freely abandon the desire to expect and maintain prepandemic normalcy for its own sake. These strategies of resistance to a politics of white neoliberal expectation are transferable as knowledge. There are some aspects of living according to crip time that can instruct us about what care labor and its distributions would look like postpandemic if we were to radically reconsider the future of "normalcy" and renarrate care work in just and liberating ways. As a writing time, crip time offers a liberating alternative for renarrating desires for able-bodied normalcy in which one no longer "needs any help."

There is a reality of disabled embodiment that must be accepted and neither subverted nor erased. The temporalization of the everyday that suspends the desires for and expectations of normalcy—as a "cripping" of everyday time—has, as I think of it, two modes: one of *synchronicity* and the other of *diachrony*.[46] This difference between everyday time and temporalizing the everyday to accommodate one's disabled bodymind[47] became less substantial during the pandemic, with so many of us finding ways to accommodate sickness or its prevention, manipulating ways to socialize against the isolation and confinement, shifting the necessary labors and work as it was now disconnected from traditional work spaces and work schedules.

Crip survivorship depends on a labor-intensive *synchronicity*—a carefully cripped reproduction of the day-to-day—in which the pace of organic life is fundamentally slower, requires respite, is flexible and inflexible in ways that radicalize the demands of neoliberal accelerationism in which we "ought" to have been working harder and faster, expecting a return on investments quickly and expediently, but just cannot. The synchronicity of crip time suspends those familiar but exhausting expectations of "efficient outcomes." It is the consistent routine to yield basic survivorship, as in the need to toilet, to medicate, to sleep, to eat. In this cripped temporalization, one cannot afford to "skip a dose" or "rush routine" when it comes to self-care or in the arranging for care; it is the importance of not only being "on time" but giving things "enough time."

Yet, in another way, this synchronicity is separate yet parallel to *diachronous* time, the time of interruptions, what philosopher Emmanuel Levinas might call "the event of non-indifference."[48] This is the labor that comes with the abrupt stops and jolts, creating immense friction with the everyday, just as it can be with the steady onset of new symptoms that finally need urgent attention, or with the sudden need for a hospital stay.

The synchronous and diachronous labors in their necessity are also sites of potential trauma, which, when one is already rendered isolated and alienated, is inescapable, and can be long-lasting, without any future remediation. These parallel temporalities have distinct labors and distinct burdens, not always properly narrated as a kind of *necessary political knowledge* even though it is just that. In order to have a place in the world that is habitable and survivable, there is already a wealth of crip knowledge generated to relieve those conditions of unnecessary suffering caused by the assumption that by simply existing, you are too burdensome.

So perhaps what follows from this are new and alternative expectations that crip time is a valid form of survivorship, and that any labor in the name of help must always carry a real "prosthetic effect."[49] This could mean a source of advocacy and solidarity in creating environments of consent over paternalism. This might look like (1) a right of refusal in the producing and reproducing of care work, something that Federici noted does not happen in unwaged and waged service labor; (2) timely care that provides relief rather than "escape" from the need for help, such as access to free and appropriate medication; (3) assistance and aid as a part of the infrastructure rather than resourced as a commodity or through charity; and (4) incorporation of institutionalized, rewardable strategies for reporting and maintaining consensual care correction, important for both the synchronicity of effective caretaking routines as well as for the diachronous shifts of labor and resources required for antiableist collective care.

If we can thus reframe "pandemic time" as "crip time," the bearing of risk can shift from those affective and emotional costs that are often unreciprocated, often without the right of refusal as Federici described it, to directing new kinds of survivorship and community care. Why must it still be that we are seen as "nagging bitches, not as workers in struggle"?[50] Without genuinely reframing and renarrating care labors, we can expect that what will come to pass is more unnecessary, useless suffering, endemic to a future that is not resistant to the desires for a "new normal" or to the pervasive want to "return to normal."

I AM WORTHY. WE ARE WORTHWHILE: THOUGHTS IN PLACE OF A CONCLUSION

As a final note, again from Piepzna-Samarasinha's *Care Work*, "Cripping the Apocalypse, 'Abled People: Time's Up'":

> It breaks my heart every time . . . [if] movements got together about ableism, there is so much we could win—movement spaces where elders, parents, and sick and disabled folks . . . could be present—strength in numbers! We could create movement spaces where people don't "age out" of being able to be involved after turning forty or feel ashamed of admitting any disability, Crazyness, or chronic illness. We could create visions of revolutionary futures that don't replicate eugenics—where disabled people exist and are thriving, not . . . where winning the rev[olution] means we don't exist anymore because everyone has health care.[51]

As I complete writing this, it is a year and a half since the pandemic was named as such in downstate New York.[52] The Delta variant of COVID-19 is again normalizing familiar political fault lines along the helpless/helpful binary and unfairly burdening some in ways that are fully life-threatening while, at the same time, claiming protection for rights and freedoms given to already privileged others (see figure 3). We continue to evade responsibility for both the just distribution of resources and, accordingly, decisions about who has access to protections from unnecessary, sustained harms.

So, in that way, while I will not submit that all grief is equal, I can add that grief is not a competition.[53] In fact, the range of "loss" experienced by so many marginalized, multiply disabled people will take years of labor to fairly frame into meaningfulness and shape into new discourses, far removed from the whitewashed illusions of a "new normal" and the caricatures of helper-heroes. I keep thinking through the urgency of the problem of "useless suffering," burdening those already considered burdens, the urgency of needed care embedded in the alienation and isolation that ties together disparate experiences of grief and loss. For me, one of the most urgent concerns moving forward is what constitutes the meaning of *burdensomeness* itself. This is especially so if underwritten and intersected by so many other forms of dismembering phenomena and vicious white neoliberal infrastructures of care.[54]

While considering that the future in the wake of a global pandemic is labor-intensive, we should not succumb to toxic positivity and wishful thinking. Instead, I suggest we ought to be guided by the insights of Critical Disability Studies as a critique of neoliberal phantasms of whitewashed, neutral, and benign savior technologies. I remain dissatisfied with the deeply ableist cultural imaginary that wishes still for a return to the "before

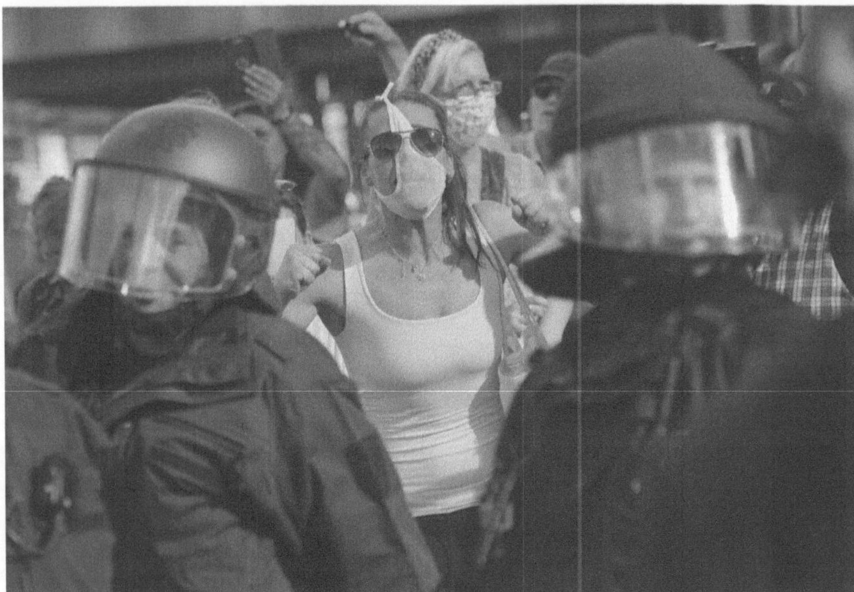

Figure 8.3 A white woman standing behind police in riot gear, with others protesting the government requirement for wearing masks. She is wearing sheer underwear on her face. Her fists are raised, and mouth is open, shouting. ***Credit: https://www.vice.com/en/article/pkbybg/germany-far-right-covid-decade-of-hate SEAN GALLUP/GETTY IMAGES***

COVID"—from businesses defending and reclaiming their revenue, to safety-sacrificing labor practices of the largest of corporations, generating unthinkable profit over the past two years—so much, in fact, that billionaire CEOs can realize their fantasies of going to space. I would not be the first to note the bizarrely timely release in 2020 of the Netflix film *I Care a Lot*, providing an accurate yet seemingly satirical reflection of how easy it is to win out and get one over on the sick and disabled, despite the justifications that the narrative of the film is "just a playful fiction."[55]

The labor of future-directed thinking is real and worthy when it is revolutionary. As Federici suggested in 2012, "communities of care . . . aim at socializing, collectivizing the experience of illness, pain, grieving and the 'care work' involved . . . to reclaim and redefine what it means to be ill, to age, to die. . . . These efforts need to be expanded."[56] There is so much to reclaim if we first abandon the romanticized need for normalcy. Yet that is the antiableist challenge of this future labor if we are to genuinely take up the call, in the words of Havi Carel, that "illness" is a prompt "to philosophise."

BIBLIOGRAPHY

Abdelmahmoud, E. "Netflix's 'I Care a Lot' Isn't the Movie It Thinks It Is." *BuzzFeed News*, February 26, 2021. Accessed October 23, 2021. https://www.buzzfeednews.com/article/elaminabdelmahmoud/netflix-i-care-a-lot-review-rosamund-pike.

Baker, R. K. "Our Divisions Evoke the Civil War, but So Do Mass COVID-19 Deaths among Caring Strangers." *USA Today*, January 4, 2021. Accessed March 27, 2021. https://www.usatoday.com/story/opinion/2021/01/04/covid-like-civil-war-dying-among-strangers-out-of-sight-column/4114439001/.

Carel, H. "Pathology as a Phenomenological Tool." *Continental Philosophy Review* 54 (2021): 201–17. http://doi.org/10.1007/s11007-021-09538-9.

Chappell, B. "Coronavirus: New York Creates 'Containment Area' around Cluster in New Rochelle." NPR, March 20, 2020. Accessed October 23, 2021. https://www.npr.org/sections/health-shots/2020/03/10/814099444/new-york-creates-containment-area-around-cluster-in-new-rochelle.

Cohen-Rottenberg, R. "What It Means to Be a Help Object." *Disability and Representation: Changing the Cultural Conversation*, September 3, 2013. Accessed October 23, 2021. http://www.disabilityandrepresentation.com/2013/09/03/what-it-means-to-be-a-help-object/.

Cook, I. "Who Is Driving the Great Resignation?" *Harvard Business Review*, September 15, 2021. Accessed October 23, 2021. https://hbr.org/2021/09/who-is-driving-the-great-resignation.

De Cruz, H. "The Case for Alternating In-Person and Virtual Conferences." *Blog of the APA*, July 15, 2021. Accessed October 23, 2021. https://blog.apaonline.org/2021/07/15/the-case-for-alternating-in-person-and-virtual-conferences/?fbclid

=IwAR3QUPWbzbxQPTuFz8yAsKsw__LbYeqcBtVoIjik3DvLMPwJsxVPKEnOr1o.

Federici, S. *Re-enchanting the World: Feminism and the Politics of the Commons*. Oakland, CA: PM Press, 2019.

———. *Revolution at Point Zero: Housework, Reproduction & Feminist Struggle*. Oakland, CA: PM Press, 2012.

Fox, M. "Lost Jobs, Less Pay, No Childcare: A Year into the Pandemic, Women Are Not OK." CNBC, March 1, 2021. Accessed October 23, 2021. https://www.cnbc.com/2021/03/01/from-jobs-to-pay-the-coronavirus-pandemic-has-hurt-women.html.

Gold, M., and E. Shanahan. "What We Know about Cuomo's Nursing Home Scandal." *New York Times*, August 4, 2021. Accessed October 23, 2021. https://www.nytimes.com/article/andrew-cuomo-nursing-home-deaths.html.

Hall, K. Q. "Reimagining Disability and Gender through Feminist Disability Studies: An Introduction." In *Feminist Disability Studies*, ed. K. Q. Hall. Bloomington: Indiana University Press, 2011.

Hamraie, A., and K. Fritsch. "Crip Technoscience Manifesto." *Catalyst: Feminism, Theory, Technoscience* 5, no. 1 (2019): 1–34.

Kingett, R. "The Pandemic Made My Industry Accessible, I'm Worried about Going 'Back to Normal.'" *The Unwritten*, June 16, 2021. Accessed October 23, 2021. https://www.theunwritten.co.uk/2021/06/16/the-pandemic-made-my-industry-accessible-im-worried-about-going-back-to-normal/.

Kisner, J. "The Lockdown Showed How the Economy Exploits Women. She Already Knew." *Anarchist Agency*, February 21, 2021. Accessed October 23, 2021. https://www.anarchistagency.com/critical-voices/jordan-kisner-the-lockdown-showed-how-the-economy-exploits-women-she-already-knew/.

Levinas, E. "Diachrony and Representation," 97–120. In *Time and the Other* [*and additional essays*], trans. R. Cohen. Pittsburgh, PA: Duquesne University Press, 1982/1987.

———. "Useless Suffering," 156–67. In *The Provocation of Levinas: Rethinking the Other*, ed. R. Bernasconi and D. Wood. New York: Routledge, 1988.

McRuer, R. "Compulsory Able-Bodiedness and Queer/Disabled Existence," 369–78. In *The Disability Studies Reader*, fourth edition, ed. L. J. Davis. New York: Routledge, 2013.

———. "No Future for Crips: Disorderly Conduct in the New World Order; or, Disability Studies on the Verge of a Nervous Breakdown," 63–78. In *Culture—Theory—Disability: Encounters between Disability Studies and Cultural Studies*, ed. A. Waldschmidt, H. Berressem, and M. Ingwersen. London: Transcript Verlag, 2017.

McRuer, R., and L. Johnson. "Cripistemologies: Introduction" and "Proliferating Cripistemologies: A Virtual Roundtable." *Journal of Literary and Cultural Disability Studies* 8, no. 2 (2014): 127–47, 149–69. http://doi.org/10.1353/jlc.2014.0013.

McWade, B. "Recovery-as-Policy as a Form of Neoliberal State Making." *Intersectionalities: A Global Journal of Social Work Analysis, Research, Polity, and Practice* 5, no. 3 (2016): 62–81.

Milbern, S., and P. Berne. "My Body Doesn't Oppress Me, Society Does." Barnard Center for Research on Women. May 9, 2017. Accessed October 23, 2021. https://www.youtube.com/watch?v=7r0MiGWQY2g.

Mitchell, D., S. Snyder, and L. Ware. "Curricular Cripistemologies: The Crip/Queer Art of Failure," 37–53. In *Das Geschlecht der Inklusion*, ed. J. Budde, S. Offen, and A. Tervooren. Berlin: Verlag Barbara Budrich, 2016.

National Governors Association. "Governors' Role in Promoting Disability Employment in COVID-19 Recovery Strategies." SEED Memo, March 23, 2021. Accessed October 23, 2021. https://www.nga.org/center/publications/governors-role-in-promoting-disability-employment-in-covid-19-recovery-strategies/.

Piepzna-Samarasinha, L. L. *Care Work: Dreaming Disability Justice*. Vancouver: Arsenal Pulp Press, 2018.

Reynolds, J. M. "'I'd Rather Be Dead Than Disabled'—The Ableist Conflation and the Meanings of Disability." *Review of Communication* 17, no. 3 (2017): 149–63. http://doi.org/10.1080/15358593.2017.1331255.

———. "Infinite Responsibility in the Bedpan: Response Ethics, Care Ethics, and the Phenomenology of Dependency Work." *Hypatia* 31, no. 4 (fall 2016) DOI:10.1111/hypa.12292.

Samuels, E. "Six Ways of Looking at Crip Time." *Disability Studies Quarterly* 37, no. 3 (2017). http://doi.org/10.18061/dsq.v37i3.5824.

Scuro, J. *Addressing Ableism: Philosophical Questions via Disability Studies*. Lanham, MD: Lexington Books, 2017.

———. "Helpfulness and Helplessness in the Time of COVID-19." Public Philosophy Network Short Talks #2. May 28, 2020. Accessed October 23, 2021. https://www.youtube.com/watch?v=iAnz2LfFBQc.

———. "The Loss of Meaningful Work." *Blog of the APA*, December 11, 2019. Accessed October 23, 2021. https://blog.apaonline.org/2019/12/11/the-loss-of-meaningful-work/.

Scuro, J., with S. Tremain. "Dialogues on Disability: Shelley Tremain Interviews Jennifer Scuro." *Biopolitical Philosophy*, March 17, 2021. Accessed March 27, 2021. https://biopoliticalphilosophy.com/2021/03/17/dialogues-on-disability-shelley-tremain-interviews-jennifer-scuro/.

Shapiro, J. "Walking a Mile in Their Patients' Shoes: Empathy and Othering in Medical Students' Education." *Philosophy, Ethics, and Humanities in Medicine* 3 (March 12, 2008). http://dx.doi.org.molloy.idm.oclc.org/10.1186/1747-5341-3-10.

Springer, S. *Fuck Neoliberalism: Translating Resistance*. Oakland, CA: PM Press, 2021.

Stern, A. "Forced Sterilization Policies in the US Targeted Minorities and Those with Disabilities—and Lasted into the 21st Century." Michigan University's Institute for Healthcare Policy and Innovation. September 23, 2020. Accessed March 27, 2021. https://ihpi.umich.edu/news/forced-sterilization-policies-us-targeted-minorities-and-those-disabilities-and-lasted-21st.

UN Women. "COVID-19 and Its Economic Toll on Women: The Story behind the Numbers." September 16, 2020. Accessed April 8, 2021. https://www.unwomen.org/en/news/stories/2020/9/feature-covid-19-economic-impacts-on-women.

Wattles, J., A. Sangal, M. Macaya, M. Mahtani, M. Wagner, and A. Vogt. "Jeff Bezos Goes to Space." CNN Business, July 20, 2021. Accessed October 23, 2021. https://www.cnn.com/business/live-news/jeff-bezos-space-flight-07-20-21/h_18cd45be2dd95b74cd7e4f6dc670dbef.

Weise, J., with É. Young. "Disabled Queer Poet Jillian Weise Upends Ableist Assumptions in Cyborg Detective." Interview with *3:AM Magazine*, September 26, 2019. Accessed October 23, 2021. https://www.3ammagazine.com/3am/disabled-queer-poet-jillian-weise-upends-ableist-assumptions-in-cyborg-detective/.

"Why COVID-19 Has Impacted Black Women So Badly." *Huffington Post*, February 25, 2021. Accessed October 23, 2021. https://www.huffpost.com/entry/why-covid-19-has-impacted-black-women-so-badly_n_602afa11e4b06d64049f1826.

Williams, Z. "Fat-Shamers Have Felt Enabled by COVID, and It's Hard to Fight Back." *Guardian*, March 7, 2021. Accessed October 26, 2021. https://www.theguardian.com/commentisfree/2021/mar/07/fat-shamers-have-felt-enabled-by-covid-and-its-hard-to-fight-back.

Winter, D. "Iconic George Floyd Mural at Cup Foods Vandalized Again, Called 'Satan's Mural.'" *Minnesota Reformer*, October 5, 2020. Accessed October 24, 2021. https://minnesotareformer.com/briefs/iconic-george-floyd-mural-at-cup-foods-vandalized-again-called-satans-mural/.

Zak, D. "American Exceptionalism Was Our Preexisting Condition." *Washington Post*, July 23, 2020. Accessed October 23, 2021. https://www.washingtonpost.com/lifestyle/style/american-exceptionalism-was-our-preexisting-condition/2020/07/22/158f5ab0-cabc-11ea-91f1-28aca4d833a0_story.html.

NOTES

1. H. Carel, "Pathology as a Phenomenological Tool," *Continental Philosophy Review* 54 (2021): 201–17, http://doi.org/10.1007/s11007-021-09538-9, para. 2. Carel goes on to note ambivalence about the use of the term "forceful invitation": "[On] the one hand, it is an urgent call, a demand for reflection. On the other hand, it remains optional. Not all who are invited will, or ought to, respond reflectively to illness. I suggest that illness plays an active role as a motivation for, or entry gate into, philosophy. The role of illness is not limited to that of a passive object of phenomenological scrutiny. Rather, I propose that illness, and pathology more generally, can be developed into a phenomenological method in their own right."

2. D. Mitchell, S. Snyder, and L. Ware, "Curricular Cripistemologies: The Crip/Queer Art of Failure," in *Das Geschlecht der Inklusion*, ed. J. Budde, S. Offen, and A. Tervooren (Berlin: Verlag Barbara Budrich, 2016), 48.

3. I want to thank Lauren Duffy, Kevin Timpe, Sara Protasi, Alisa Jahns, Devonya Havis, Sumati Deutscher, and especially Anna Gotlib for their assistance in the drafting of this chapter.

4. As of the time of this original drafting, there was an estimated 2,759,685 deaths from COVID-19 worldwide, 558,497 in the United States, the largest number of

deaths than any other country. I have not included any information about the Delta variant in this statistic.

5. Which in hindsight was also connected to a toxic positivity in which well-meaning people often suggested that I "look on the bright side" and how "everything will be okay," often told to me as way of "helping." I had little mental and emotional resource to be able to resist the way this kind of help that wasn't really help, exacerbating my stress and underlying illness. I would find out in April 2021 postoperatively that I had had uterine cancer and significant endometriosis.

6. See, for example, Joel Michael Reynolds's analysis, "'I'd Rather Be Dead Than Disabled'—The Ableist Conflation and the Meanings of Disability," *Review of Communication* 17, no. 3 (2017): 149–63, http://doi.org/10.1080/15358593.2017.1331255.

7. See the report by Bill Chappell, "Coronavirus: New York Creates 'Containment Area' Around Cluster in New Rochelle," NPR, March 20, 2020, accessed October 23, 2021. https://www.npr.org/sections/health-shots/2020/03/10/814099444/new-york-creates-containment-area-around-cluster-in-new-rochelle.

8. These are claims I make in my book, *Addressing Ableism: Philosophical Questions via Disability Studies* (Lanham, MD: Lexington Books, 2017). I cite here the idea of Western somatophobia as foundational to ableism, as referenced by Kim Hall in summarizing Susan Wendell's work, (see K. Q. Hall, "Reimagining Disability and Gender through Feminist Disability Studies: An Introduction," in *Feminist Disability Studies*, ed. K. Q. Hall (Bloomington: Indiana University Press, 2011), 5.

9. The association between shame, despair, and unemployment, as I describe it here, is not exactly the same as what has led what has been dubbed the Great Resignation of 2021. My concern outlined is for the way in which disability connotes that one is also unemployable, and therefore, must expect to remain unemployed or, at least underemployed and underpaid. The history of labor abuses and the exploitation of the job market when it comes to sustained employment of disabled people is complex and we see an analogous problem for wage labor workers and nonunion service workers suddenly called "essential" during the pandemic. For an account of this Great Resignation, see Ian Cook's report "Who Is Driving the Great Resignation?" *Harvard Business Review*, September 15, 2021, accessed October 23, 2021, https://hbr.org/2021/09/who-is-driving-the-great-resignation, and for more on the issue of employment on disabled people and communities, see National Governors Association, "Governors' Role in Promoting Disability Employment in COVID-19 Recovery Strategies," SEED Memo, March 23, 2021, accessed October 23, 2021, https://www.nga.org/center/publications/governors-role-in-promoting-disability-employment-in-covid-19-recovery-strategies/.

10. See R. McRuer, "No Future for Crips: Disorderly Conduct in the New World Order; or, Disability Studies on the Verge of a Nervous Breakdown," 63–78, in *Culture—Theory—Disability: Encounters between Disability Studies and Cultural Studies*, ed. A. Waldschmidt, H. Berressem, and M. Ingwersen (London: Transcript Verlag, 2017).

11. R. McRuer "Compulsory Able-Bodiedness and Queer/Disabled Existence," in *The Disability Studies Reader*, fourth edition, ed. L. J. Davis (New York: Routledge, 2013), 371–72.

12. Carrie Sandahl, who coins the term "crip" as both a verb and as a critical strategy, gives testimony that (quoted in R. McRuer and L. Johnson, "Proliferating Cripistemologies: A Virtual Roundtable," *Journal of Literary and Cultural Disability Studies* 8, no. 2 (2014): 167. http://doi.org/10.1353/jlc.2014.0013):

> [In] 2003, when I coined the verb "to crip," as I needed a verb to describe the strategies that crip, queer, solo autobiographical performance artists use in their work to critique not only mainstream communities but disability and queer communities as well. My original definition was that cripping "spins mainstream representations or practices to reveal able-bodied assumptions and exclusionary effects. Both queering and cripping expose the arbitrary delineation between normal and defective and negative social ramifications of attempts to homogenize humanity, and both disarm with a wicked humor, including camp."

13. See Simon Springer's *Fuck Neoliberalism: Translating Resistance* (Oakland, CA: PM Press, 2021) for one of my favorite critiques of neoliberalism—as a market-based system that is ideologically, economically, and politically driving the idea of normalcy as also compulsory able-bodiedness. An application of this critique as it is attached to recovery is by Brigit McWade, "Recovery-as-Policy as a Form of Neoliberal State Making," *Intersectionalities: A Global Journal of Social Work Analysis, Research, Polity, and Practice* 5, no. 3 (2016): 62–81.

14. Helen De Cruz applies Kingett's argument to make the case for keeping philosophy conferences accessible in her post, "The Case for Alternating In-Person and Virtual Conferences." *Blog of the APA*, July 15, 2021, accessed October 23, 2021, https://blog.apaonline.org/2021/07/15/the-case-for-alternating-in-person-and-virtual-conferences/?fbclid=IwAR3QUPWbzbxQPTuFz8yAsKsw__LbYeqcBtVoIjik3DvLMPwJsxVPKEnOr1o.

15. R. Kingett, "The Pandemic Made My Industry Accessible, I'm Worried about Going 'Back to Normal,'" *The Unwritten*, June 16, 2021, accessed October 23, 2021, https://www.theunwritten.co.uk/2021/06/16/the-pandemic-made-my-industry-accessible-im-worried-about-going-back-to-normal/, para. 12–16.

16. From Weise in an interview with Élan Young, "Disabled Queer Poet Jillian Weise Upends Ableist Assumptions in Cyborg Detective," interview with *3:AM Magazine*, September 26, 2019, accessed October 23, 2021, https://www.3ammagazine.com/3am/disabled-queer-poet-jillian-weise-upends-ableist-assumptions-in-cyborg-detective/, para. 24. Cy goes on to explain the cyborg versus the "tryborg":

> A cyborg's body is technology. So I'm a cyborg because my leg is a computer. And here the tryborgs—my name for nondisabled people who theorize about cyborgs—will want to argue: "No, you have a fake leg." There's nothing fake about it. It's my leg. And it's my computerized part. If my leg starts buzzing, which it does occasionally, to communicate with me, and then dies, that changes

my body and the trajectory of my day. So in essays for *Granta* ("Common Cyborg") and the *NYT* ("Dawn of the Tryborg"), I return the word *cyborg* to disabled people. We were the first cyborgs, and we are the ones integrating our bodies with tech" (para. 6).

17. I borrow this language from A. Hamraie, and K. Fritsch. "Crip Technoscience Manifesto," *Catalyst: Feminism, Theory, Technoscience* 5, no. 1 (2019): 1–34: "Disabled people design our own tools and environments, whether by using experiential knowledge to adapt tools for daily use or by engaging in professional design practices. Crip technoscience conjures long histories of daily adaption and tinkering with built environments" (para. 9).

18. A draft of this paper was given as a virtual lecture as part of the lecture series BPL Philosophy in the Library, "The Burdens of Labor and Imagining Future Care Communities," hosted by the Brooklyn Public Library and the Brooklyn Public Philosophers, May 20, 2020. I also want to note that disability scholar and activist Stacey Milbern died the day before I gave the talk and so I dedicate this piece to her and her legacy. For more on Milbern, see her in conversation with Patty Berne, "Crip Bits," a video series hosted by *Sins Invalid*, "My Body Doesn't Oppress Me, Society Does," Barnard Center for Research on Women, May 9, 2017, accessed October 23, 2021, https://www.youtube.com/watch?v=7r0MiGWQY2g.

19. See, for example, Dan Zak's article "American Exceptionalism Was Our Preexisting Condition," *Washington Post*, July 23, 2020, accessed October 23, 2021, https://www.washingtonpost.com/lifestyle/style/american-exceptionalism-was-our-preexisting-condition/2020/07/22/158f5ab0-cabc-11ea-91f1-28aca4d833a0_story.html.

20. See J. Wattles, A. Sangal, M. Macaya, M. Mahtani, M. Wagner, and A. Vogt, "Jeff Bezos Goes to Space," CNN Business, July 20, 2021, accessed October 23, 2021, https://www.cnn.com/business/live-news/jeff-bezos-space-flight-07-20-21/h_18cd45be2dd95b74cd7e4f6dc670dbef.

21. I discuss material from this section in a video short posted by Public Philosophy Network, "Helpfulness and Helplessness in the Time of COVID-19," Public Philosophy Network Short Talks #2, May 28, 2020, accessed October 23, 2021, https://www.youtube.com/watch?v=iAnz2LfFBQc.

22. There is significant concern in the scholarship about this desire to help the "less fortunate," the "poor," and the "disabled," because vulnerable persons become subsumed into an abstract class. This desire effects a dangerous form of othering. See for example, J. Shapiro, "Walking a Mile in Their Patients' Shoes: Empathy and Othering in Medical Students' Education," *Philosophy, Ethics, and Humanities in Medicine* 3 (March 12, 2008), http://dx.doi.org.molloy.idm.oclc.org/10.1186/1747-5341-3-10, in which she states, "The most extreme form of othering is scapegoating, or the way in which individuals and groups pursue wholeness and reject the frightening or impure elements of themselves (such as vulnerability to illness and death) by projecting them out onto others" (para. 15).

23. R. K. Baker, "Our Divisions Evoke the Civil War, but So Do Mass COVID-19 Deaths among Caring Strangers," *USA Today*, January 4, 2021, accessed March

27, 2021, https://www.usatoday.com/story/opinion/2021/01/04/covid-like-civil-war-dying-among-strangers-out-of-sight-column/4114439001/

24. Much gratitude for Macias's permission to use this post. For an expanded account, see: https://aworkstation.com/you-think-coronavirus-is-scary-this-nurses-viral-post-shows-its-worse-than-you-imagine/.

25. I borrow this term from Emmanuel Levinas and his essay "Useless Suffering" (in *The Provocation of Levinas: Rethinking the Other*, ed. R. Bernasconi and D. Wood [New York: Routledge, 1988]), which he describes is not the suffering itself that I might experience in its intimacy and absurdity, distinct from the pains I might suffer but that come with reward, but the magnified horror of the suffering of the Other because of the indifference to the other's suffering, most notable in the atrocities of the twentieth century, "despite these cruelties, because of these cruelties" (159).

26. Cohen-Rottenberg cites her conversation with her friend Julie Rose: "If you offer me help and I don't accept it, I'm an ungrateful, ungracious asshole. It doesn't matter is what you are offering me is useful or not. It doesn't even matter if what you are offering me might be life threatening to me" (R. Cohen-Rottenberg, "What It Means to Be a Help Object," *Disability and Representation: Changing the Cultural Conversation*, September 3, 2013, accessed October 23, 2021. http://www.disabilityandrepresentation.com/2013/09/03/what-it-means-to-be-a-help-object/, para. 4).

27. Take, for example, the practice of forced sterilization; see: A. Stern, "Forced Sterilization Policies in the US Targeted Minorities and Those with Disabilities—and Lasted into the 21st Century," Michigan University's Institute for Healthcare Policy and Innovation, September 23, 2020, accessed March 27, 2021, https://ihpi.umich.edu/news/forced-sterilization-policies-us-targeted-minorities-and-those-disabilities-and-lasted-21st.

28. I would additionally argue, as tied to compulsory able-bodiedness, these assumptions about who needs help extends to the current revised versions of fat-shaming that came with increased Coronavirus risk. See Zoe Williams, "Fat-Shamers Have Felt Enabled by COVID, and It's Hard to Fight Back," *Guardian*, March 7, 2021, accessed October 26, 2021, https://www.theguardian.com/commentisfree/2021/mar/07/fat-shamers-have-felt-enabled-by-covid-and-its-hard-to-fight-back: "It is not a tragedy, it is just those less important people. It is not the cruel and random hand of fate, it is a sound moral outcome—undisciplined people who had it coming got it. . . . Fat-shaming never owns its agenda . . . [and] because it never speaks its name, the fat-hate, you can never argue against it" (para. 3–5).

29. McRuer and Johnson, "Cripistemologies," 132.

30. S. Federici, *Re-enchanting the World: Feminism and the Politics of the Commons* (Oakland, CA: PM Press, 2019), 178, 180–81. I want to thank Élaina Gauthier-Mamaril for a good discussion about being "shipwrecked" in relation to my career in academic philosophy.

31. Federici, *Re-enchanting the World*, 111. My reading of Federici is selective because of the outstanding issues of Federici's analysis in *Beyond the Periphery of the Skin* (Oakland, CA: PM Press, 2020), which does not seem to carry the same (and arguably works against) insights she offers in other texts. See one critique by Cory

Austin Knudson: http://www.full-stop.net/2020/05/28/reviews/cory-austin-knudson/beyond-the-periphery-of-the-skin-silvia-federici/?fbclid=IwAR3iqGjAS-jl3wxxAcjufKQN6feZUzclqFnuuerr2JG8GT-94XC_OHPCSFk.

32. See Kisner's account originally published by the *New York Times Magazine*'s subsection "The Future of Work": "The Lockdown Showed How the Economy Exploits Women. She Already Knew," *Anarchist Agency*, February 21, 2021, accessed October 23, 2021, https://www.anarchistagency.com/critical-voices/jordan-kisner-the-lockdown-showed-how-the-economy-exploits-women-she-already-knew/.

33. S. Federici, *Revolution at Point Zero: Housework, Reproduction & Feminist Struggle* (Oakland, CA: PM Press, 2012), 19.

34. UN Women, "COVID-19 and Its Economic Toll on Women: The Story behind the Numbers," September 16, 2020, accessed April 8, 2021, https://www.unwomen.org/en/news/stories/2020/9/feature-covid-19-economic-impacts-on-women

35. Federici, *Revolution at Point Zero*, 20.

36. This is discussed at length in chapter 4 on Precariousness in my book *Addressing Ableism*.

37. Federici, *Revolution at Point Zero*, 101).

38. See "Why COVID-19 Has Impacted Black Women So Badly," *Huffington Post*, February 25, 2021, accessed October 23, 2021, https://www.huffpost.com/entry/why-covid-19-has-impacted-black-women-so-badly_n_602afa11e4b06d64049f1826; and M. Fox, "Lost Jobs, Less Pay, No Childcare: A Year into the Pandemic, Women Are Not OK," CNBC, March 1, 2021, accessed October 23, 2021, https://www.cnbc.com/2021/03/01/from-jobs-to-pay-the-coronavirus-pandemic-has-hurt-women.html.

39. See Ellen Samuels's "Six Ways of Looking at Crip Time," *Disability Studies Quarterly* 37, no. 3 (2017), http://doi.org/10.18061/dsq.v37i3.5824. I want to thank my friend and colleague Sara María Acevedo for her support and collegiality in working out these ideas for the classroom.

40. L. L. Piepzna-Samarasinha, *Care Work: Dreaming Disability Justice* (Vancouver: Arsenal Pulp Press, 2018), 69.

41. Piepzna-Samarasinha, *Care Work*, 71.

42. See my "Dialogues on Disability" interview on the blog, *Biopolitical Philosophy*, March 17, 2021, accessed March 27, 2021, https://biopoliticalphilosophy.com/2021/03/17/dialogues-on-disability-shelley-tremain-interviews-jennifer-scuro/.

43. Federici, *Revolution at Point Zero*, 104.

44. Samuels, "Six Ways of Looking at Crip Time," para. 1.

45. Samuels, "Six Ways of Looking at Crip Time," para. 21.

46. In Joel Michael Reynolds's discussion of response ethics, also drawing from the work of Emmanuel Levinas, in the context of caring for his grandfather, describes the "dialectic of embodied response in dependency work," accounts for three "moments" similarly, "leveling, attention, and interruption." With attention, "I prepare, at least provisionally, for the response of the other. A constant shift from leveling to attention is the mark of an exemplary dependency worker," and with interruption, "whether attentive or not, one will encounter moments of *interruption*. . . . Moments of interruption puncture the leveling of the other and condition the necessity of attention."

("Infinite Responsibility in the Bedpan: Response Ethics, Care Ethics, and the Phenomenology of Dependency Work," *Hypatia* 31, no. 4 (fall 2016): 785).

47. I am following Piepzna-Samarsinha's use of the term, especially as it can assist in the critique of the manipulative desire for normalcy:

> "Mainstream ideas of 'healing' deeply believe in ableist ideas that you're either sick or well, fixed or broken, and that nobody would want to be in a disabled or sick or mad bodymind. . . . but . . . abound that disabled and sick folks are sad people longing to be 'normal,' that cure is always the goal, and that disabled people are objects who have no knowledge of our bodies. And deep in both the medical-industrial complex and 'alternative' forms of healing that have not confronted their ableism is the idea that disabled people can't be healers" (*Care Work*, 103).

48. This idea of the diachronous I borrow from Levinas's ethical metaphysics, particularly when he describes in "Diachrony and Representation" (in *Time and the Other* [*and additional essays*], trans. R. Cohen [Pittsburgh, PA: Duquesne University Press, 1982/1987]) an awareness and onset of an ethico-existential "election," "an awakening to the other person . . . irreducible to knowledge, . . . it is a non-indifference to the other" in which, is not 'pure rupture' but akin to "adventure" or "intrigue" of the 'degradation' in the perceived 'unity of time' upon the demand of the ethical (108, 118–19).

49. I have termed this as a kind of 'prosthetic effect' and discuss my experience in interview with Shelley Tremain.

50. Federici, *Revolution at Point Zero*, 16.

51. Piepzna, *Care Work*, 128.

52. It is worth noting the reporting about how the now-resigned New York State governor hid the impact of the coronavirus on nursing home and assisted living facility residents in an effort to look "proactive" in managing the pandemic. See M. Gold and E. Shanahan. "What We Know about Cuomo's Nursing Home Scandal," *New York Times*, August 4, 2021, accessed October 23, 2021, https://www.nytimes.com/article/andrew-cuomo-nursing-home-deaths.html.

53. I want to credit my former colleague Dennis Ryan for this important insight.

54. It is worth noting the murder of George Floyd in May 2020 and the impact it had on disabled communities, especially disabled communities of color. The reaction by the white, ableist conservative mainstream was, as to be expected, exemplified by the vandalizing of the George Floyd mural with red spray paint exclaiming, "'FUCK . . . COMMIES & SATAN." See Deena Winter's report "Iconic George Floyd Mural at Cup Foods Vandalized Again, Called 'Satan's Mural,'" *Minnesota Reformer*, October 5, 2020, accessed October 24, 2021, https://minnesotareformer.com/briefs/iconic-george-floyd-mural-at-cup-foods-vandalized-again-called-satans-mural/.

55. As one reviewer notes, "it gives the impression that the film was never seriously interested in exploring elder abuse, just in using it as a vehicle to get to a hollow thriller that exploits American culture's obsession with scammers. . . . Plus, the timing of the movie is really unfortunate. It is not *I Care a Lot*'s fault that it is arriving in

the middle of a global pandemic that has brutally exposed the neglect with which we treat older adults. Nor is it the movie's fault that it premiered a couple of weeks after a documentary on Britney Spears' conservatorship sparked calls for a reckoning about the ways the current system takes power from people with disabilities" (E. Abdelmahmoud, "Netflix's 'I Care a Lot' Isn't the Movie It Thinks It Is," *BuzzFeed News*, February 26, 2021, accessed October 23, 2021, https://www.buzzfeednews.com/article/elaminabdelmahmoud/netflix-i-care-a-lot-review-rosamund-pike, para. 11–12).

56. Federici, *Revolution at Point Zero*, 125.

Chapter 9

Boundaries of Democratic Life in a Time of Pandemic

Alexios Alexander[1]

The COVID-19 pandemic took hold of my imagination in March 2020, the day before our campus shut down for six months. A student who had just finished collecting the newly completed midterm exams abruptly sneezed all over them. I promptly dismissed class, reminding everyone of the precautions they should take, and gingerly walked to my office with the exams extended a foot from my body. This, it turns out, would be one of the *least* troubling moments of the next nineteen (and counting) months. The precautions I mentioned were only those commonly known to keep students from spreading regular colds and the flu to each other. No one in my class had worn a mask, of course, as the CDC and WHO had not yet called for this public health measure. Indeed, public health messaging stated both that there was (fear of) a dire mask shortage and that masks were not efficacious against COVID-19 anyway—a contradictory set of reasons and messages, even if coordinated to prevent the buying of surgical and N-95 masks. Even after public health officials began to offer coherent, consistent guidance, the American public could neither unite nor agree on fundamental issues wrought by the pandemic. Social trust was clearly broken at the very worst time. The pandemic, at best, has offered us the most confusing of times, and at worst, the most desperate and painful of times. Ubiquitously, it has been deeply disruptive.

Disruptions, however, open space and time for reflection; they provide critical distance from normality. Routines are destroyed, or at least delayed, and our thoughts and actions operate without the bannisters[2] that otherwise help us sleepwalk through days, weeks, seasons, years. COVID-19, to put it mildly, ruptured the orders and logics that typically govern our lives. Buses no longer transported children to school, and day care was canceled. Millions of jobs were lost permanently, some temporarily, and others moved fully or partially online. Hospitals were overrun; hugging and indoor socializing became dangerous. Various boundaries were transgressed and redrawn, contested and ignored, deemed meaningless or existentially necessary.

For some, the threat of the virus reaffirmed the need for solidarity in the face of interlocking crises of global reach. Family members moved in together to save money, help those who were laid off, and assist with child and elder care. Neighbors went grocery shopping for the elderly and immunocompromised. Workers went on strike to protest unsafe workplace conditions. Activists harangued politicians about super-spreader conditions in prisons and nursing homes. Funerals and weddings were canceled or moved online for the sake of the attendees and their relationship circles. People routinely wore masks and kept their physical distance from others, especially when indoors; those with symptoms further isolated themselves, staying quarantined and separated from partners and family members for weeks at a time. This response to the pandemic understands boundaries and bindings as sources of freedom and flourishing, as the way to coordinate collectively for the common good. Inscribed in this response is the understanding that limits, obligations, and communal relations are preconditions for public freedom rather than impediments to it.

For others, however, the putative threat of the virus instead confirmed the dangers of authority (whether state, media, or scientific) and bolstered self-reliance to the point of self-destruction. Gun sales skyrocketed, as if gunslinging cowboys might shoot the virus dead—or worse, as if some citizens viewed their neighbors as threats to poach the goods being hoarded. Many would protest mask-wearing mandates by toting their guns around, unconcerned by the viral threat but armed and ready to defend their "freedom"—specifically, the "freedom to ignore" these legally and socially imposed boundaries to their actions. In contrast to stores with a "customers must wear a mask" policy, some stores *prohibited* customers from wearing masks. This response to the pandemic understands boundaries and bindings as a cure worse than any disease—the very source of unfreedom.

Did the pandemic create this divide, or were these sociopolitical and philosophical fault lines already with us? If the latter, what latent subjectivities, what forms of life, were already in operation? How did we think ourselves bound and free before? Will the pandemic rupture routinized thought and action so that we might think and act anew, bound up with each other in service of collective flourishing? This chapter will explore how understandings of freedom and human flourishing relate to the dynamics of boundaries, in the hope that understanding them better might allow for their reconfiguration.

FORMS OF LIFE IN A TIME OF PANDEMIC

Widespread "antimask" rallies amid a pandemic are curious events.[3] Even so, the collective, public burning of protective masks performed at many of these rallies seems stranger yet.[4] As a form of protest, rallies might be readily explained as a rational political strategy to motivate public officials to enact the policy preferences of the protestors.[5] Mask burning, however, describes behavior befitting a ritual—a novel, perhaps spontaneous ritual, but a ritual nonetheless. Political rituals are quite common, of course—we might think of the pledge of allegiance to the flag, singing the national anthem, taking an oath of office, or, alternatively, the burning of the national flag. Of these examples, the oath taking, pledge of allegiance, and singing of the national anthem are rituals meant to solidify the social bonds of affection around patriotism, whether from state officials or those they represent. These rituals spring from forms of life meant to affirm belonging to that imagined community known as the nation. The ritual of burning, on the other hand, functions as a form of expression against, if not the nation per se, then the actions of the state. In an important sense, some portion of the people whom the state is meant to represent feel harmed, unheard, and angry at the state's betrayal of certain principles, of the violation of some set of boundaries. Indeed, protest can itself express a form of solidarity, flowing from a form of life where those who care for their community or even for those across the country or across the globe demand justice on their behalf. Sometimes, defiance is the most patriotic action one can take; other times, defiance betrays a lack of concern for others, expressing instead a focus on oneself and the capacity to act as one wishes.

If the burning of the flag (or a draft card, to name another example) represents the defiance of a political order that has betrayed its citizenry by drafting them into an unjust war, of what dominating political and social order does the mask-burning ritual represent defiance? Masks are material limits, boundaries that contain the space of breath and in doing so guard against the virus. In destroying the very material that limits the spread of COVID-19, what boundaries do the protestors hope to erase? One 2021 mask-burning rally in Pittsburg was promoted as the "Americans for Freedom Rally."[6] Interestingly, at this rally, mask burning *and* singing the national anthem were performed. What understanding of freedom is sought here? What kind of patriotism? To answer such questions, it is helpful to recognize that these were not the only set of pandemic protests that erupted with the clarion call for freedom from oppressive state action.

In the summer heat, months into year one of the COVID-19 pandemic, the murder of George Floyd ignited mass nationwide protests on a scale not seen since the assassination of Dr. Martin Luther King Jr. Of course, while the police killings of unarmed men and women of color certainly lit the spark for these protests, the meaning of the protests cannot be reduced to one police killing or even the fraught issue of policing. Indeed, the time in which these protests and the "antimask" protests arose was not only a time of a public health crisis, but also a time of interlocking political, social, and economic crises. Both sets of protests expressed outrage, specifically in relation to state action, and both were concerned with the violation of a certain understanding of freedom and state oppression—yet two more dissimilar understandings of each term could not likely be imagined.

How might we understand these two distinct expressions of political agency and mobilization within the body politic in a time of pandemic? In what ways might their respective political demands shed light on contested understandings of freedom and human flourishing? How is it that both sets of protests concern the principle of freedom and the injustice of oppression, yet seem so disconnected in their respective understanding of those realities? How does this contrast relate to broader social and political divisions over fundamental questions of how to live together in a democratic republic? To answer such questions, it helps to back up a bit.

The novel coronavirus known as COVID-19 breached our borders long before it disturbed our collective awareness. Many had already died in China and Italy by then, and this upsetting news had certainly percolated through the body politic. But for most Americans, only after an emergency travel ban was issued and lockdown orders began did it seem to register that this global pandemic was also local. Suddenly it became *our* pandemic. From mass graves and overrun hospitals to the more mundane suffering of Zoom fatigue, from the loneliness of locking down and deprivation of human touch to the fear of job losses or dangers of working on the front lines, many surely proclaimed: "Life as we know it has ended." For many, a quick succession of questions followed suit: How long must we endure this? When might we "return to *normal*"? Yet these questions arose among diverse populations, infusing disparate assumptions into the meaning of the terms "life," "we," "know," and "normal." For the life that we know, the life that is normal, is never an abstraction, but always finds meaning in the web of concrete relationships in which our specific lives are lived.

In his twentieth-century text *Philosophical Investigations*, renowned philosopher of language Ludwig Wittgenstein[7] illustrates how the meaning of a word varies depending upon the specific context of its use. For example, the bark of the tree has a different meaning from the bark of the dog. Moreover, these contexts usually take place in the stream of conversations among people who share various norms, practices, worldviews—in specific *forms of life*.[8] In many instances, what is meaningful to some is nonsensical to others. If you have not played or heard of the game Monopoly, you are unlikely to grok the phrase, "Do not pass go, do not collect $200," as it would not have been part of a language game you had played given the forms of life in which you have lived. Similarly, who you are, your social location, and, more broadly, the forms of life in which *your* life is situated drastically alter the referential meaning of words like "normal"—and indeed, of entire phrases like, "Life as we know it has ended." Yet how can we understand the various contexts and forms of life that give meaning here? What *might* one mean by "my life" in the language games where such meaning is in question? What are the boundaries that give meaning to your life and what in the web of life is *yours*?

You might answer by listing the people in your life, the property you own, the work you do, the family you belong to, where you live—a set of particularities that situate you in space, in time, and in relationship to others with whom you identify. Of course, your life is also bound up with the lives of others ("No man is an island," as the saying goes—sorry, Robinson Crusoe). You share and situate your life in various communities. Boundaries demarcate our web of relationships and commitments. Indeed, from the global community to the nation, state, city, household, and, in a time of pandemic, the "pod"—boundaries tell us how to situate ourselves. We understand ourselves as connected by and embedded within various bounded relationships: personal, familial, social, and political. These relationships generate communities, and to whom we imagine ourselves connected, who counts as part of our community, affects how we think ourselves obligated to each other.

Put another way: how we behave toward others depends upon who we think they are in relation to us—are they bound up with us, are they part of one of our communities? Or are they outside our commons and thus "on their own"? Such questions are predicated on an understanding of collective human flourishing in which my good and your good are bound up together. This is the root meaning of the term "commonwealth." The question of who is included and who is excluded in our various communities is an ongoing process, keeping alive the concern for who is cared for and on what terms. This dynamic of inclusion and exclusion, of situating relational duties, manifests in many ways. It is both social and political, as our forms of life inform how we make judgments, how we behave, and how we respond to disruptions.

Different forms of life give rise to distinct language games that give meaning to terms like "freedom" and "flourishing." These divergent understandings of freedom and flourishing have consequences. In a pluralistic society such as the United States, these consequences reflect and exacerbate long-standing political and social realities and conflicts. In a global pandemic, these consequences cascade and confront our collective awareness, exposing yet deeper origins of these forms of life in the institutions and governing logics that structure them. Such exposure presents an opportunity for social and political transformation, which in turn requires philosophical inquiry into these realities and their formation. The disruptions caused by the pandemic thus open space to reconsider our social relationships and forms of life. This time for reflection also permits space for political action—action that expresses the understandings of proper boundaries and bindings that shape identities and worldviews.

For some, COVID-19 made us recognize and affirm how we might live in community and solidarity. From this way of thinking and living, we needed to understand how we were bound up together, how we might protect rather than endanger those within our sphere of concern, and how our sphere of concern should include everyone and anyone we might affect with our actions. This form of life concerns itself with a social contract in which ignoring the needs and well-being of others is akin to harming one's own life. This involves thinking about what promises we have made to one another, even if only implicitly. Examples of this abound: giving up your bus seat for an elderly or infirm person, holding the door for someone imminently approaching, helping someone up who has fallen down. These are communal logics in operation. Covering one's mouth when coughing or sneezing, not invading someone's personal space or yelling at them—betraying these basic forms of decency can and do become existential threats during a pandemic. The shift from basic decency to lifesaving measures drastically alters the stakes of social obligation for those who already attend to the lives of others as part of their own communal concern.

For others, however, the virus brought with it different needs. It demonstrated the danger of the "Other," the need to resist authority (state, scientific, media), and the need to reassert individualism, even against a communal threat. Insofar as this way of thinking and living considers others, the focus is on Other(s) as threat and those in positions of authority as threat. Strangely, an egocentric form of life in which one's agency is at the fore often drastically concerns itself with the agency of others and what they might do. Paranoia, rather than conceptions of a public good, can become the primary mode of thinking about others and institutions.

BOUNDARIES OF FREEDOM AND FLOURISHING

In these divergent responses, what ways of thinking and acting predominate? How do these contrasting ways of life understand freedom? It is worth noting that regardless of how they are conceptualized, freedom and flourishing are fundamentally connected. Insofar as one desires and values freedom, this principle is instrumentally linked to other values and ends. These values and ends vary, but however they are selected or ranked, they ultimately amount to a notion of a life worth living. Freedom permits one to pursue life that is *good*, a life that is not *merely* life, not *bare* life, but a life of meaning (this likely calls to mind the famous "life, liberty, and the pursuit of happiness" language of the Declaration of Independence, and for good reason). Although freedom is a principle that can be valued for its own sake, the principle of freedom worth preserving and fighting for is necessarily, if often implicitly, the freedom to live a life worth living.

One way to think about the meaning of terms like "freedom" and "flourishing" is to consider not only what freedom and flourishing mean and require, but also *whose* freedom and flourishing is in question. Often the question of who is included or excluded is itself an indicator of the very meaning of freedom and flourishing to those drawing the boundaries. This makes it crucial to ask: Is it my freedom that is in question, or your freedom, or our freedom? Whose flourishing or good is of concern? If it is not only *my* freedom or well-being that is in question, then who else is included? The context of the question, in turn, often implicates who (or what) else is involved in this question—who or what are the *obstacles* to freedom and who or what *enable* freedom. Moreover, how does my freedom and my flourishing relate to the freedom and flourishing of others?

One influential answer to such questions came from the seventeenth-century English philosopher Thomas Hobbes, a thinker quite familiar with plague and pandemic. Hobbes wrote at a time when epidemics afflicted England so regularly that the frontispiece of his 1651 magnum opus *Leviathan* depicts, below the famous image of the body politic–as-Leviathan, a quarantined city, with near empty streets traversed only by soldiers and two plague doctors.[9] The fear of danger from infectious disease in this image parallels the fear of chaotic danger Hobbes sees in the natural state of human beings: that is, the chaos of a war of all against all, with each individual person operating at cross-purposes with every other, unless an all-powerful sovereign steps in and instantiates law and order. Human beings, in this image, are mostly understood as threat, and ultimately their conflicting passions must be curtailed by sacrificing natural liberty for limited civil liberties (as delineated by the sovereign alone).

In this powerful political vision, Hobbes's *Leviathan* is one of the earliest and most influential depictions of the human world as a world of atomized individuals.[10] Indeed, the very concept of an "individual" human being, existing and understood separately from the relations and communities in which he or she is embedded, was quite novel. Hobbes (in)famously defines the natural world of human beings as one of discrete bodies in motion, each body a bundle of appetites and aversions moving the body toward or away from what attracts or repels. For Hobbes, to be naturally free or at liberty consisted in the ability of a given body to move toward that which it desires and away from that which it seeks to avoid.[11] Freedom is always and everywhere a desire of atomized individuals. To take away someone's natural liberty, in this conception, is merely a matter of constraining their ability to move as they wish (though interestingly, this constraint must be physical, as Hobbes does not recognize psychological obstacles as impediments to freedom).[12] From a certain Hobbesian perspective, public health measures in a pandemic requiring quarantine, lockdown, physical distancing, and the barring of entry to certain spaces (bars, restaurants, etc.) would be fundamentally understood as restricting individual natural liberty.

Furthermore, Hobbesian freedom and liberty draws no distinction between what is desired and what is good (and therefore worth desiring and pursuing). What I desire is that which I call "good," that which repels me I merely label "bad," and liberty and license are conflated. The one caveat for Hobbes is that self-preservation is a fundamental natural drive or desire, and so one might err insofar as one is drawn toward that which is destructive of that fundamental end.[13] Otherwise, on this understanding, you cannot err, you cannot love nor hate the wrong things; pursuit of your desires and pursuit of your good is always the same endeavor.

Against this individualistic pursuit, encountering other bodies in motion poses a constant threat and potential obstacle. Atomized individuals are each moving and acting in ways that might conflict, that might deprive each other of the liberty to fulfill their respective desires—including the ultimate denial of liberty in death. The state of nature, it turns out, is also a state of war. Fear of death and this state of atomized competition—"a war of all against all," for Hobbes—are the problems of social action he seeks to solve through the social contract.[14] One might join a political community, then, for the security of a world in which those obstacles to your desires are singularly codified in law. When entering the social contract, natural liberty is sacrificed for both self-preservation and some measure of civil liberty (that which the law permits). In terms of exercising the freedom of natural right, stores with "masks required" policies and stores with "masks prohibited" policies have equal standing. For Hobbes, therefore, only the Leviathan—the centralized, all-powerful state—can dictate which of these policies would constitute justice and which would be unjust. This, of course, would lead most Leviathans to prevent infectious disease from spreading, and in so doing to keep its side of the bargain in the social contract. The antimask protesters, insofar as their protestations concern freedom, inherit only part of the political lineage from Hobbes's vision. These protesters operate in line with his anthropology and the concomitant natural right to exercise their power, yet they are less interested in leaving the state of war to enter a social contract that sacrifices this Hobbesian liberty for order and security. They wish to keep the power to do

whatever they desire, irrespective of how it affects their fellow citizens, *and* they wish the state to stay out of this conflict.

For Hobbes, agreeing to be bound by absolute rule of law, to be bound to the Leviathan, is a deal worth making. The Leviathan, to be clear, is his name for the sovereign, and though the sovereign must have absolute power, the form of government might be a monarchy, an aristocracy, or even a parliamentary system. The key is that the state instantiates law and order, protecting individual actors from each other, so that they may move freely according to the boundaries drawn by the state, by being bound to the social contract that circumscribes where one can and cannot move and act. Even if the antimask protesters reject the social contract and its bargain, they embrace the Hobbesian understanding of atomistic bundles of desire fighting for their natural right to do as they wish.

For these protesters, as with Hobbes, the locus of political freedom is in that private sphere where the state does not interfere with one's ability to move and act as one desires. Metaphysically, Hobbes also thinks one is free to break the law and suffer the consequences, even if those consequences are likely to either imprison or kill you. In this political vision, the laws of the state primarily operate as an obstacle to and constraint on freedom, even if in service of a broader good—a life *otherwise* unbound and yet protected against the interference of others. That is, to live a life free of the interference of others, to be free to act as you wish, while understanding the clear legal consequences, that is the best deal you can get in this vision. This is a political order that gives rise to forms of life where bare life and fear of death subside and make way for a better, more meaningful life—even if atomized and understood at the individual level of meaning-making and pursuit. It is also a way of life where concern for self takes priority, and insofar as relationships matter, it is in how they interfere with the self. Above all, it is the relationship to the state that cannot be ignored.

For eighteenth-century Swiss philosopher Jean-Jacques Rousseau, political freedom has an altogether different meaning, as does human flourishing. It is in his philosophical lineage that the George Floyd protesters and mutual aid networks can be understood as fighting for an altogether different vision of political freedom and flourishing. For Rousseau, man is "born free, but everywhere he is in chains."[15] Hobbes's picture of the human world as replete with competitive, conflict-ridden interactions among alienated egoists is accurate, for Rousseau—but importantly, not as our *natural* way of being. This egoistic, antagonistic image is true to *what we have become* in society, shaped by the norms, mores, and laws that structure alienating and *unfree* forms of life. In this understanding, the two sets of protests offer us glimpses into different ways of being, different forms of life, that we can choose to become or not. According to Rousseau, our human nature might well have meant for us to be simple, solitary creatures, but since we are highly adaptable and influenced by our environment, there is no "going back" to a time before society began to shape how we live and act.[16] We can transform ourselves because laws and norms are our creations; though we craft the chains, we can just as well craft the keys to unlock them. We see this manifest in the varied responses to the crises of the pandemic worldwide and the subsequent variance in death tolls. Many polities could have done better, and we can all yet do better. The running human toll in this existential accounting illustrates who we have been and continue to be in this pandemic, socially and politically.

Whereas for Hobbes, freedom is bound up with one's private desires and individual possibilities for action, for Rousseau, freedom is a public affair, with one's own freedom bound up with the communal and political relationships that make its exercise possible. In his understanding of the social contract, each citizen is "forced to be free" by submitting to the democratically derived laws of the state. By active participation in the democratic processes that shape what the law is, each citizen helps form the "general will" to which they are all obligated. This duty, this obedience, is itself the expression and manifestation of political freedom. Importantly, the democratic process involved and the "will" that results must not be an aggregation of individual wills (this would be what Rousseau terms the "will of all"); instead, each citizen must properly understand that the "will" they are shaping is that which serves the common good.[17] In this political vision, submitting your will to *every*-one is at once submitting it to *no*-one, and your freedom and good is inextricably bound up with the freedom and good of all. In this way of life, democratically passing a national mask mandate and a national vaccine mandate would have been instantiations of freedom and the means to serving the common good.

The "will of all" might be thought of as exemplified by an opinion poll—which, by definition, is an aggregation of individual wills. This explains why, in such polls, you often see contradictory results: As an aggregated desire, the people want to increase the funding of programs and services provided to them but decrease their tax contribution. Americans want to reopen "the economy" from a particular lockdown, but also to reduce COVID-19 case counts. If the "will of all" is pursued in such instances, no one receives what they desire, as they are not thinking about themselves in relation to others (or, if they are, they think of themselves in contradistinction from others). When the "will of all" fails to deliver, atomized individuals aggregate to form factions, or a "corporate will." Oil companies receive subsidies that increase their profits but harm the environment and foster climate change, private prisons profit from caging citizens, corporations who use prisoners to produce their goods benefit from the nearly free labor, a delivery service where workers' bathroom breaks are penalized—such a list of examples, sadly, could continue for pages upon pages. During the pandemic, this was evident in the propping up of various industries (cruise ship, airline, etc.) rather than a focus on the physical safety or even job security of the workers in those industries. Hospitals, losing money because of the cessation of elective surgeries, laid off nurses and staff at the very moment that the need for nurses and staff skyrocketed because of COVID-19 patients. The pursuit of the corporate will leads to neither freedom nor flourishing but merely adds another form of conflict and competition, another power struggle divorced from public freedom and the common good. Instead, a way of life might be pursued that understands cooperation, interdependence, sacrifice, trust, and reciprocity. This requires forms of life and language games where the meanings of freedom, oppression, and flourishing are shared.

Not only do the visions from Hobbes and Rousseau consider the meaning of freedom and human flourishing, but each offers a particular social contract. A contract, of course, is an agreement wherein and whereby the parties involved make binding promises. For a nation-state, this is an implied and implicit agreement springing from forms of life that are predicated upon it. The promising involved in such a social contract, however, does not merely bind you to those to who have also made this promise, but also enacts a kind of self-binding; you bind yourself—that is, your future self—to act or not act (whatever the case may be) in some predetermined way. To some, this stability, this ordering of future actions, might seem a form of unfreedom, a restriction of liberty. And while it is indeed a restriction, a limit, a binding and a boundary, the question of how this promise relates to freedom is not so simply determined but depends on the language games at play in a particular form of life. For Hobbes, the constraints of submitting to the Leviathan permit the possibility of pursuing desires with the security against interference from others provided by law and order. For Rousseau, to bind yourself in a certain way is a form of freedom. This form exists only as a democratic way of life, informed by an active citizenry who imagine each other bound up together. To promise to adhere to a boundary set by law, arrived at democratically, is to manifest a self-relation and relationship to others and to the state that promotes freedom and flourishing.

The above represent but two philosophical lineages that still permeate the language games of political and social meaning-making in the United States. Hobbes and Rousseau are merely two of many influential sources of meaning and boundary drawing for political and social forms of life. However, their use of a term such as a "freedom" exists alongside the use by other influential thinkers whose conceptions of such terms share what Wittgenstein called a "family resemblance." For example, in libertarian forms of life, most prominent is perhaps a Lockean nose, even if a Hobbesian chin is discernible. That is, in a particular language game, the use of the word "freedom" might relate most closely to Locke's theorizing of the origin and significance of property rights and the private ownership that flows from those rights. In another context, "freedom" might resemble the Hobbesian state of nature, in which all desires are equally licensed and freedom is the ability to be unbound, unrestricted in pursuit of these desires. Thus, we can identify, if not their precise lineage, at least the "family resemblance" displayed in contemporary forms of life and language games.

This identification implicates questions such as: How do we relate to ourselves, to others, to the state—what boundaries and bindings are involved? Is the resemblance to a family of ideas that sees human beings as atomized and self-sufficiently able to pursue their own good, if only the obstacle of other people and the state get out of the way? Or is the resemblance to a family of ideas where the common good is the proper end that orients how we move and act, and where there is an ongoing pursuit of *expanding* the boundaries delineating who is included in the commons. Considering such questions helps contextualize the political and social realities that came to the fore during the pandemic. It is to the pandemic and these forms of life that we now return.

CONCLUSION: A VIRUS, TOO, RELIES ON OTHERS

The spread of COVID-19 in the United States has respected neither boundaries nor borders. A virus does not discriminate but is an equal opportunity invader. The nature of a virus is to spread itself, to replicate and enter any host whose defenses fail to stop it. Viral movement is mediated by such hosts, and so to persist, to stay in movement, a virus relies on others. This reliance entails only that the hosts do not defend themselves and each other but instead act just as they normally do, feeling free to ignore the invasion. The profound asymmetry of death and suffering experienced in the United States across racial and class lines, therefore, does not owe its reality to virology alone. Neither is the virus responsible for the racial, gender, and class lines along which duties of care work have been drawn (whether relating to spheres of medical care, childcare, or elder care). Rather, the social and political responses to the virus and the social and political realities that existed before its arrival account for these disparities. The virus harms the vulnerable the most, but social and political stratification accounts for the asymmetries both in death and illness—for such stratification determines who is protected and who is ignored, who is pushed into harm's way and considered "on their own." Ruth Wilson Gilmore, prison abolitionist and geography scholar, refers to these asymmetries as the "distribution of vulnerability to premature death."[18] Certain forms of life support the ossification of these asymmetries;

other forms of life challenge and seek to transform the institutions, policies, and norms that entrench them. It is to these contrasting forms of life and their respective language games that we now turn.

A nation, as the influential political scientist Benedict Anderson writes, is an imagined community.[19] So, too, are smaller communities. Consider, for example, the relationship to self, other, and boundaries involved in the creation of the quarantine "pod." A pod is the name given to two or more households who arrange to exclusively share space, air, and duties of care. The concept of the quarantine pod arose during the pandemic to meet social needs and maintain relational bonds while still staying bound to public health guidelines and goals. The concept might be thought akin to the metaphor of "two peas in a pod," as it connotes shared values that bind people to one another, as well as captures the image of protection and flourishing shared among those who are bonded. The mutual trust and boundedness of the pod arrangement serves to obligate pod members to one another. Deciding to pod (and, in turn, choosing a particular pod) is therefore to demarcate a boundary. This boundary is drawn and agreed upon by those who agree to the compact that governs the pod. Some in the pod might have to sacrifice more than others, just as others perhaps require more assistance. In their boundedness, pod members can move and live freely with each other. Pod members understand that to act in accordance with limits, to respect boundaries, borne of shared purpose, yields greater freedom. This, of course, is a microcosm of how a healthy body politic and its social compact might function. The important difference, of course, is that the bonds of affection that connect those in a pod are based upon personal knowledge and familiarity—only family and friends need apply. To extend this care to the imagined community beyond the familiar is the task of politics. Civic friendship means caring for all those whom your political bodies govern, as they are all inextricably bound up with you in pursuit of a common good.

Perhaps now is a good time to return to the two sets of pandemic protests discussed at the outset. While no mass gathering is monolithic, the contrasting ways of life that inform the understandings of freedom and oppression in these two sets of protests is palpable—we can recognize from which family of ideas each protest descends.

Of the millions of protesters who gathered to speak out against the police killing of George Floyd, many came out specifically on behalf of those they did not and could not know; they came to fight for the stranger. Reports of the diversity of the crowds reflect that while many protested for their own family and neighbors, many were also protesting for those members of the broader imagined communities within and across the nation. These mass protests, despite often involving thousands of people, were not found to be super-spreader events, as masks and physical distancing were the governing norms. Indeed, the threat of spreading the virus came most often when the police would "kettle" the crowds, as well as from the arrests and imprisonment of protesters.

The freedom demanded in these protests is tied to a sense of communal flourishing. Communal flourishing, in this vision, requires freedom from the violence of the state. As such, the political demands were first and foremost that the police stop killing men and women of color, because Black Lives Matter. Protesters who make this demand understand that once Black lives matter, the boundaries of who is included in the public good are significantly expanded. Such demands were coupled with complementary demands for housing the unhoused, for stopping evictions in a pandemic—for those state policies that, in serving the good of those who have been neglected, foster both freedom and flourishing for all. In addition to protests, the organization and mobilization of people in communities across the country sprung from and increased awareness of the needs and vulnerabilities of those often neglected by the state. To a degree, this extension of care to the larger community has taken the form of mutual aid in addition to political demands. This mutual aid is often a stopgap measure, put in place by concerned community members in the absence of sufficient governmental action. Community refrigerators, food pantries, and other distribution mechanisms have become the Band-Aids covering those preexisting wounds exacerbated by the pandemic. As the pandemic has underscored the fissures in American society, political demands have also gained strength. The essential workers on whom the professional managerial classes depend live lives of precarity and increased vulnerability. In this pandemic context, renewed political support for racial justice, unions, strikes, demands to increase to the minimum wage, Medicare for All, and so forth, offer the possibility of reorienting our imagined community and reframing our relationships and obligations. These possibilities are imagined and demanded by citizens enacting a democratic way of life, in search and in service of the common good.

In contrast, the symbolism expressed in the ritual mask burning at various "antimask" rallies is, quite clearly, a message of defiance. The mask itself is the object that *others* told you to wear, whether the state, your boss, the store manager where you shop, your neighbor, or the many imagined residents of the United States. As an act, burning the mask destroys the object that represents the perceived oppression; it is the physical representation of tyrannical control, of unfreedom. Antimask protesters appear to consider the mask, despite its more obvious public health function, as an oppressive, socially required garment, the wearing of which is expressive of a socially mandated role. One might consider this ritualistic burning alongside other such instances of political protest.

During the Vietnam War protests, flags and draft cards were sometimes burned with other perceived items of oppression, such as dish soap. If the burning of flags and draft cards were objections to compulsory participation in the death and violence of war, the burning of dish soap is connected to the socially mandated role that required women to be homemakers. This role and way of life dictates what range of choices should or should not be pursued based on one's gender identification. In short, the nature of the oppression being protested here is the attempt to structure both individual and collective ways of life in a specific way. The freedom sought in opposing the politically mandated role of military service and the socially mandated role of the dutiful housewife is freedom from killing others while risking one's own life, on the one hand, and freedom from patriarchal control of identity and fundamental life choices, on the other. The Vietnamese, in one example, are included within the boundary of those who deserve to live. In the other example, the rigid boundary of what intimate and family relations look like can be redrawn to bind people to each other in new and evolving ways. These political rituals, unlike those of the antimaskers, are not pitted against the value and flourishing of other lives, but instead express new imaginings of what is conducive to flourishing and whose lives should indeed matter politically and socially. This invites the question: What politically and socially mandated roles are antimakers resisting in the name of "freedom"?

The function of the mask, insofar as it relates to a socially mandated role, is to acknowledge and respect the mutual dependence and shared vulnerability of life during a pandemic. Of course, the pandemic did not create this interdependence and reciprocal vulnerability, but merely highlighted and made more pronounced the visibility and consequences of how our lives affect each other. To the extent that there is freedom in refusing to wear a mask, it is the freedom to ignore how one's most basic choices and actions can harm the individual and collective good of other people; it is the freedom to be atomized and separate, a world unto oneself. This self-enclosure draws the boundary of the commons at the boundary of the skin-encapsulated ego, befitting a society of competitive egoists. This a freedom tied to the good of isolation and separateness. The atomized body in motion that sees others as obstacles, that sees one's own desire as infringed upon when the good of others interferes—this resembles the Hobbesian agent.

This defensive, enclosed way of life is also reflected in (now former) President Trump's emergency closing of borders to noncitizens only, alongside his administration's messaging around the so-called China Virus or Wuhan Virus. The Hobbesian move here is to attach the fear of an infectious disease to very particular human beings who themselves become dangerous and threatening; this, in turn, creates space for an authoritarian leader of "law and order" to step in and protect against the dangerous people who pose this threat. To the xenophobe, every problem looks like an Other, and ignoring the science of how a virus spreads complements the focus on other human agents as the sole locus of danger and concern. Indeed, this emergency closing of borders was coupled with a short deadline for citizens to rush back to the United States, overcrowding airports and risking the mass spread of the virus. In 2020, some Trump rallies, antimask rallies, and, perhaps most infamously, the Trump administration's celebration of the Supreme Court nomination of Amy Coney Barrett were COVID-19 super-spreader events. This latter event represents the flip side of projecting danger of a virus onto the Other, whether that other is from abroad or of a different race or even socioeconomic class: It is to think oneself invulnerable.

Such destructive ways of being are not purely partisan, however. The disregard for the particularly vulnerable was evident in how governors, mayors, and state legislatures alike abandoned those without stable housing as well as those in prisons and nursing homes. The hesitancy to "lock down" and the concomitant eagerness to "reopen" cut across party lines, as did decisions to close parks while reopening for-profit gyms. The decision to close safe outdoor public spaces (which, in a time of cabin fever borne of lockdown, are especially liberating and good for people) while opening indoor spaces where heavy breathing and close proximity are the norm only makes sense from a standpoint where capital accumulation matters more than human life and human needs. Insofar as local and state governments felt constrained to act against those needs and in service of "the economy" (another imagined boundary that ignores the people who work and live in it), the federal government's failure to act is clear. However, the forms of political and social life that similarly valued a "return to normalcy" were those reflected in policies generating precarity and death for warehouse workers, nurses, restaurant servers, and others deemed both "essential" and "heroes"; their good and their freedom were considered, if at all, as a worthy sacrifice so that those safely ensconced at home could fulfill their own needs and desires.

A successful public health response to a pandemic requires coherence and unity at three levels: public health capacity and response, state action, and social acceptance and cooperation. Although failures were rampant on all fronts, many of the political and social failures arose from forms of life and particular understandings of principles like freedom that betrayed the fundamental trust and communal bonds imagined in most social contracts. The only exception is the kind of social contract that Hobbes offers, which is a contract of mutual indifference (though in this vision, at least the Leviathan, if no one else, is looking out for the welfare of the entire *demos*). Forms of life that internalize such a political imagination view both the state and other people as mere obstacles to desire being fulfilled, and so are always sources of disturbance and oppression. Little wonder, then, that firearm sales rapidly rose at the start of the pandemic and firearms accompanied many of those who burned masks in protest.

In contrast, mutual aid stations sprung up in the George Floyd protests and in anarchist enclaves such as the one established in Portland, Oregon. Social trust, coordination, and the meeting of needs were the values tied to the demands for freedom from oppression. State violence and state failure to meet the needs of the people were the harms to the social fabric being contested, and that informed the communal responses. Of course, this response can also support "the economy," as the boundary between the economic and the political can be drawn to unite rather than to separate the two spheres. Indeed, the economic, political, and social spheres are bound up together. Workers are also residents of communities, and their livelihood and safety are inextricable from a proper pandemic response.

I fondly recall visiting Greece as a child and realizing that my uncle, who was a small business owner, would close his shop down for several hours each day around lunchtime—to be with his family for lunch and a nap. Twice a week, the store stayed closed for the day. Of course, this was not a problem for his business because his competitors were doing the very same. This was not a problem for overall economic activity—people did not consume less but merely coordinated when to shop for their goods so that time with family, time for a nap, was integrated into their lives alongside the shopping tasks. Importantly, such a way of life does not begin and end its understanding of "the good" with a singular individual's desires. It understands freedom and the common good as inclusive of as many members of the nation as possible. Those who demand the United States share its vaccine supply across the globe widen this imagined community further still: to all with whom we share our human existence. The pandemic yet holds possibility for us all, if only we reconfigure the boundaries between us in ways better suited to a "COVID-19 world"—a world whose flourishing is irreversibly and increasingly interdependent.

NOTES

1. I would like to acknowledge and thank Anna Gotlib for her helpful feedback and for organizing this volume. I am grateful to David Kaib for his insights and thoughtful engagement with my work. Lastly, I offer my deep appreciation and thanks to my partner, Bajeera McCorkle, without whom this and many other accomplishments would not be possible.

2. "Thinking without bannisters" is a phrase used by political theorist Hannah Arendt and the title of a recent collection of her essays and letters.

3. The “antimask” rallies might also be called the “antilockdown” rallies, as seemingly any protective public health measures mandated or recommended by state or health authorities were objected to in these protests.

4. From Idaho to Pennsylvania to Arizona to Florida, these mask-burning rituals are still occurring over one year into the pandemic.

5. There might be other, less rational motivations that might be at play, of course—especially those rallies that took place in locations where there were no mask mandates nor strict lockdown measures. For some, perhaps the motivation was to express anger at those who informally judge or seek to influence whether (or not) masks are worn by their fellow Americans.

6. Liz Reid and Katie Blackley, “Demonstrators in Pittsburgh Chant ‘Burn Your Mask’ and ‘Impeach Wolf’ in Protest of Coronavirus Restrictions,” WITF, March 20, 2021, https://www.witf.org/2021/03/20/demonstrators-in-pittsburgh-chant-burn-your-mask-and-impeach-wolf-in-protest-of-coronavirus-restrictions/.

7. Wittgenstein’s legacy as one of the most significant philosophers of the twentieth century is beyond dispute, even if challenges and debates remain in how to characterize his particularly idiosyncratic body of philosophical work and its influence.

8. Ludwig Wittgenstein, *Philosophical Investigations*, trans. G. E. M. Anscombe (Oxford, UK: Wiley- Blackwell, 2009).

9. Thomas Poole, “Leviathan in Lockdown,” *London Review of Books Blog*, May 1, 2020, https://www.lrb.co.uk/blog/2020/may/leviathan-in-lockdown.

10. For Hobbes, the social contract formed by atomized individuals creates one artificial person, a state authorized by these individuals, that he refers to as the Leviathan.

11. Thomas Hobbes, *Leviathan* (Oxford: Oxford University Press, 1996), 34–35.

12. Hobbes, *Leviathan*, 33–35.

13. Hobbes, *Leviathan*, 86.

14. Hobbes, *Leviathan*, 82–87.

15. Jean-Jacques Rousseau, “On the Social Contract,” in *The Basic Political Writings*, trans. Donald A. Cress (Cambridge: Hackett, 1987), 141.

16. Jean-Jacques Rousseau, “Rousseau’s Notes to *Discourse on the Origin and Foundations of Inequality Among Men*,” in *The Basic Political Writings*, trans. Donald A. Cress (Cambridge: Hackett, 1987), 104–105.

17. Rousseau, “On the Social Contract,” 204.

18. Ruth Wilson Gilmore, interview by Paul Gilroy, *In Conversation with Ruth Wilson Gilmore*, (Sarah Parker Redmond Center) https://www.ucl.ac.uk/racism-racialisation/transcript-conversation-ruth-wilson-gilmore.

19. Benedict Anderson, *Imagined Communities: Reflections on the Origin and Spread of Nationalism*, (New York: Verso, 2016).

PART IV

Pandemic, Philosophy, and Meaning

Chapter 10

More than Mere Survival

Ethical Responsibility and the Intersubjectivity of the Humanities

Claire Elise Katz

Recently I was asked by an undergraduate who was interviewing me about my research, "How is philosophy relevant to today's generation?"[1] What she meant by her question was this: How is philosophy relevant to *her* generation, the generation currently in college? Why might a current college student wish to take a philosophy course? Her question is neither unusual nor unique. The question, put more generally, applies to all generations—and has been asked certainly since I was a college student in the 1980s (and I suspect long before that).

We could frame her question this way: How might we persuade college students today that philosophy is relevant to them, even if they are majoring in business or one of the STEM fields or another discipline that appears to be wholly different from philosophy? I replied to her as I typically do to all students (indeed even nonstudents) who ask me this question: Philosophy is relevant to all generations and it has been since its inception.

Philosophy is everywhere, and most people, including young people, encounter philosophy on a daily basis. The questions it asks are embedded in both the extraordinary and the banal events of our lives. We are engaged in philosophy every time we consider an ethical decision. "What ought I do?" is a fundamental question within philosophy. I tell the students in my philosophy of education class every time they ask, "Why do we have to take X class?" that they are already engaged in a philosophical discussion about the nature of education.

When they wonder if they find something beautiful and why they think it's beautiful, they are engaged in a philosophical discussion about aesthetics. When they consider the legitimacy of a news source, they are considering questions about evidence and the nature of truth. And when they argue, regardless of their position, about whether one has a responsibility to wear a mask or if the government can mandate wearing a mask, they are engaged in a discussion about relationships of ethical responsibility between a community and individual political freedom, which is a foundational question in political philosophy.

Philosophy is also relevant to every generation. However, it might be the case that the questions that face this generation currently in college are more complicated and more difficult to address. In this chapter, I explore two ways in which the pandemic has revealed philosophy to be especially relevant to us in this historical moment.

The first addresses the myriad responses to the pandemic that reveal the tension between individual rights related to freedom and our individual and collective responsibilities to individual others and to our community. The second explores how philosophy as a subset of the humanities reveals why we care about living a life that *flourishes*—that is so much more than simply being alive—and the role the humanities play in the pursuit of that kind of life.

MORE THAN BARE LIFE

"If you want to wear a mask, go ahead. That's your choice. My choice is not to wear one." We have heard this comment or something similar since the pandemic started in spring 2020 and the view that masks would help prevent the spread of COVID-19 was put forward. On the surface, it sounds like what kids often stay to their parents: "You're not the boss of me," which if one listens carefully to that statement, reframes the parent/child relationship as a boss/employee relationship, rather than one of protector, teacher, caregiver, and so forth. The statement, usually uttered in a moment of anger or frustration because the child does not want to do whatever the parent is asking, is just another way of saying, "You can't make me [do something]."

The statements circulating about mask wearing reveal a frustration similar to the one expressed by the toddler. However, when these statements are uttered by an adult with specific political rights and obligations, a different set of issues emerges. Although there could be a general suspicion of experts, among people who are opposed to vaccines in general, the response to the COVID-19 vaccine has taken on a set of issues that, while maybe not unique, appear to be magnified by the political context in which the virus emerged. For the adult, one underlying tension in this statement is between individual freedom (both political and metaphysical) and political responsibility to the community.

Additionally, the statement, "If you want to wear a mask, that's your choice," fails to understand the science behind the mandate to wear a mask. The mask, as the science tells us, prevents more airborne particles from moving outward rather than entering. Thus, wearing a mask is less about protecting our own health, which one could argue is a personal choice (more about that shortly), than it is about protecting those around us.

Similarly, one could argue that even if wearing the mask was about protecting our own health, by not wearing a mask, individuals increase their chances of contracting and spreading the disease, thus stalling our ability to eradicate it and protect others. This, in turn, reveals that even those choices that appear to be simply personal choices about one's own health are anything but that.

In this short section, however, I wish to focus on the responsibility that we have to others. A statement that has been widely circulated on the internet, and falsely attributed to Anthony Fauci, reads, "I don't know how to explain to you that you should care about other people." The statement was originally tweeted by Lauren Morrill a week before the 2017 presidential inauguration in response to President-Elect Donald Trump's demands to dismantle the Affordable Care Act.[2] It was retweeted quickly and frequently, often without citation to Morrill.

In June 2017, six months after Morrill's original tweet, Kayla Chadwick published an op-ed in the *Huffington Post* with the title, "I Don't Know How to Explain to You That You Should Care about Other People."[3] The piece references healthcare, but its focus was the general welfare of others and our responsibility to care for them in ways that we frequently neglect. Chadwick neglected to credit Morrill's tweet as the inspiration for the title, and possibly even the framing, of her piece. Since then, the statement appears whenever there is a discussion about the fundamental obligations we have to others where that care and concern are strikingly absent.

Although I wish to give fair credit to Morrill for succinctly stating an important observation, the sentiment behind the statement has a history that long precedes her tweet. As I wrote in my 2013 book, *Levinas and the Crisis of Humanism*, reason has its limits.[4] That is for sure a difficult claim for a philosopher to write. I wrote that statement in response to a set of discussions that took place at a conference I attended on teaching philosophy to K–12 students in September 2009, not even a year into Barack Obama's presidency.

I was pushing back against the framing of ethics as an obligation that we have only when our life is not at risk. Instead, I argued that the ethical obligation remains present even when our life is at risk. We might choose to preserve our life, but that does not mean that the obligation is negated. It remains, even if we chose to protect ourselves rather than respond to the other. The fact is just that we sometimes decide to neglect, and thus fail to meet, our obligations.

Modern ethical theory has been based on a view of the self that allows for the preservation of the self to take precedence. Blaise Pascal famously stated it as, "'That is my place in the sun.' Here is the beginning and the image of the usurpation of all the earth."[5] The question that the twentieth-century French Jewish philosopher Emmanuel Levinas asked is, "How do I defend that place?" If we begin from the place of individual rights, what could you possibly say to me that would persuade me by reason to give up *my* place in the sun for *you*? And if we each continue along the road, approaching each other with the belief that our own individual place in the sun takes precedence, we are engaging in a game of ethical chicken, wondering who will cede their position to the other first.

Yet using Levinas's ethical project as a foundation, we might reframe how we approach ethical dilemmas. A traditional approach to ethics might talk about ethical decision making in terms of the self: What I ought I do? How ought I act? And these are decisions about actions that might or might not have an impact on someone else. But what if ethics were not about action? What if instead, ethics referred to the *obligation* to another, an obligation that one might say is that upon which any ethical *action* is predicated?

If ethics were about developing the self in relationship to another for whom I am responsible, whose life comes before mine, then my claim to that place in the sun is put into question from the start.[6] In a side conversation that developed shortly after the discussion at the conference described above, the example I used to illustrate this point was, not coincidentally to the focus of Morrill's and Chadwick's frustration, the ACA, which was being hotly debated at the time. The opposition to the ACA was not Trump's invention, even if Trump was doggedly determined to kill it.

Writing about this conversation later, I wondered what the ethical warrant was that would persuade someone to choose national healthcare instead of keeping his own money.[7] "Why," I asked, "would an individual accept that another's life, read here as access to that health care, is more important than, or should be privileged, over the 'right' to the money he earned? Why would he turn from his own interests to the suffering of the Other," where "Other" for Levinas refers to the ethical other, the one who is "not me" and to whom I am wholly obligated.[8] For Levinas the Other is a singular reference, identifying the other person as unique. Levinas describes the ethical obligation to the Other in a way that deviates from traditional ethical theory. He uses terms like "asymmetrical" to indicate that there is no expectation of ethical responsibility in return.

In response to this question, I wrote in *Levinas and the Crisis of Humanism*:

> In spite of claims to the contrary, it is not clear to me that reason will deliver the one correct answer. Through an appeal to economics, pragmatics, or familial obligations, reason could easily offer a justification for either claim: self-interest or care for the Other. The answer at which we arrive and the one we choose for ourselves is already conditioned by the things we value and how we understand ourselves as subjects who are rational and free. From a Levinasian standpoint, an individual will only part with her money in the service of others (without benefit to herself, e.g., a tax break) if she has first turned toward the Other—and reason does not necessarily motivate this turn to occur.
>
> The example with which I opened this introduction reveals that there is an underlying obligation that informs both possible choices—my self-interest or the needs of the Other. The stronger point to be made, however, is that these two "obligations" are not really obligations. One is assumed to be a "right," e.g., my right to my money—and the other is a responsibility for the Other, to give up some of that money in order for others simply to have health care, simply to live. That is, there is nothing in a discussion of competing rights that will turn one away from one's own rights and to the Other. Philosophy can point out the error in our ways of thinking; it can indicate that there might be other economic systems that are more just than the one we currently embrace; but it is not clear to me that philosophy necessarily turns us toward the Other. . . .
>
> As long as I see my subjectivity defined in terms of my own freedom and with my own rights as central, then any engagement with the Other will simply be a test of wills. *As long as the sovereignty of the ego remains central, then neither philosophy in particular nor a humanities education in general will be sufficient to change the heart.*[9]

Returning to our current situation of life in a pandemic, we would first need to get clear about what the mask does. Currently, many people believe that the mask protects themselves, and independently of whether they have a social obligation to reduce their risk to contract the virus, these people currently believe that they are only putting themselves at risk by not wearing a mask. In truth, however, as the science teaches us, they are putting those around them at an increased risk.

What the science tells us is that risk is greatly reduced when we all wear masks. But once we have gotten the facts straight, we still need to persuade people to care about others. From a Levinasian viewpoint, I do not think we can do that. I believe we can appeal to a level of care that is already present by explaining how the mask contributes to care for others, but I do not think we can persuade people who believe their freedom is the foundational value, subordinating any calls to consider the needs of another.

I appreciate Morrill's pithy 2017 tweet, and when others repeatedly shared her words, the credit should have been all hers. But her expression of frustration at not knowing how to persuade people to care about others is also the much older sentiment at the foundation of Levinas's ethical project, which I drew out in my 2013 book. My point here is not to engage in a battle about who had the sentiment first, but rather to address the ongoing implications of this idea for us now, long after this sentiment first captured Levinas's attention.

For Levinas, turning toward the Other will not be the result of a philosophical persuasion. As long as our ethical views remain rooted in a political philosophy that allows the ego to be central, that puts my rights above the suffering of the other, the only philosophical argument that will persuade me to care for the other is the one that still takes into account my own happiness and my own freedom—that is, my own sovereignty. As I have argued elsewhere, to get to a different place, we need a different view of the self, one that is fundamentally defined not simply as intersubjective, but a view of the self that comes into being as a subject when one is claimed ethically by the other.

The pandemic, then, reveals the underlying philosophical views that motivate how people think about their position and needs in relation to others. And although I do not necessarily believe philosophical dialogue will bring people to see why they *ought to* care about others, I do believe that understanding this particular dilemma born of reason's limitations will help us think more clearly about how and why we need to reconsider our views (and practices) of our shared subjectivities and duties to each other.

WITH A LITTLE HELP FROM MY FRIENDS

When I responded to the student who asked me about the relevance of philosophy to this generation, I gave the answer that demonstrates what philosophy can do, how philosophy works. There is obviously a side to the humanistic disciplines that has an applied value: They teach us to be literate, to think critically and creatively, to consider different perspectives, to listen, to be reflective about our own positions. In short, deep engagement with humanistic fields can provide a set of skills that can be applied to our lives, our jobs, and our hobbies.

The more difficult response is the one that suggests that there is an intrinsic value to the humanities, that engagement with the humanities provides a kind of pleasure, an intellectual joy, that is difficult to describe, but that nonetheless sustains us, often in especially difficult times. One of the loveliest lines in philosophy is Aristotle's observation in the *Nicomachean Ethics* that even with all the wealth in the world, no one would choose to live without friends. For Aristotle, philosophy itself was best done with friends. His insight is one of the first philosophical views that even the life of the mind is best achieved in the company of others, not as a solitary endeavor.

When we moved our lives indoors and away from others, Aristotle's observation revealed its truth. We enjoy the company of others not only at meals or to watch movies but also to engage in activities that appeal to the life of the mind, whether they are discussions of books or watching a play or listening to a podcast. Similarly, these activities also reveal the profoundly humanistic qualities that ground them. These activities sustain us as humans, just as food sustains us biologically.

In 2016 when I was discussing the children's book *Frederick the Mouse* with a colleague, I suggested that the book tells a wonderful story about the value of those activities we often find valueless because they do not "produce" anything.[10] Briefly, the story is about a field mouse who writes poetry while the rest of the mice in his community collect the food needed to make it through the next season.

Initially viewed as lazy and unhelpful, Frederick reads his poetry while they sit underground waiting for winter to pass. The food they collected keep the mice alive; but Frederick's poetry sustains them and helps the time pass more quickly. It makes their time waiting for the next season enjoyable—and bearable.

As a professor of philosophy, I have often found myself in the position of defending the humanities as a discipline that we pursue not only because of the applied skills the humanities develop, but also because of the sheer joy engagement with the humanities brings to those who teach and conduct research in those areas. When we watch a play, or listen to a concert, or visit an art museum, our aesthetic selves are awakened. We listen to music to soothe us, excite us, help us focus. We attend plays because they capture our attention. We visit museums because the objects they display are stunning, sometimes even in their horror, as with ancient weapons of war.

Do these activities teach us things? Yes, if we open ourselves to what they can offer. But in the moment, we partake in these activities because we enjoy them. Similarly, those of us who work in humanistic fields read and write and teach because the deep engagement with eternal questions about what it means to be human awakens our minds. These questions draw us out of ourselves and toward others; that is, they are questions that reveal fundamentally our intersubjective dimension.

As the pandemic forced so many of us fortunate enough not to put ourselves at risk but to move our lives inside, or at least to become isolated from socializing with friends, we turned toward other modes of engagement. Although I was not always engaged in face-to-face interactions with other people, the arts and humanities became a stand-in for those previous interactions. How grateful I and so many of my friends were that different arts venues were sharing their shows online—some for free and others for a small charge.

From our living room, we watched *Hamilton* and Disney. We explored national parks and museums around the world. We read more and did art projects together. I increased the time I spent walking and listened to books and podcasts while doing so. The human dimension experienced through singing, acting, dancing, artistic creation, and explorations of cultural diversity found around the world was ever present even if my interactions with real live humans had decreased substantially.

Significantly, this move into isolation also revealed the myth of independence, not only with regard to ethical obligation, as I describe above, but also our subjectivity—how we define what it means to be human—in general. Those of us living among family members did not feel this quite as much—and that situation created other difficulties with families needing help with younger children. But for people living alone, or for teenagers who could no longer engage socially with their peer group, or for elementary school kids who could not go out to play, we witnessed mental health breakdowns on a catastrophic scale.

We are not islands unto ourselves. We are fundamentally social. Although many of us are now in the throes of Zoom fatigue, using Zoom for activities that we had not originally intended, the pandemic opened up possibilities of not only staying in contact with close friends and families, but of increasing contact in ways we might not have initially imagined. For me, the best application of Zoom was allowing my seventy-nine-year-old mother, living alone in Atlanta, to join us for our Passover Seder.

Passover has always been my favorite holiday.[11] My fondest childhood memories are sitting at my grandmother's Seder table discussing politics and eating the traditional foods. Living in college towns far away from family, I've had to create my own Seder table and fill it with people about whom I care deeply and with whom I wish to share this tradition.

Although living in a community with very few Jews has been lonely in an existential way, I was so grateful to have so many friends and colleagues willing to share this tradition with me. We read the Passover story, ate the symbolic food (many were courageous enough to try the gefilte fish), drank wine, and discussed politics, academics, literature and philosophy. And we laughed—a lot.

But this year the pandemic changed all of that. My Passover Seder this year was a bit of "on the one hand" and "on the other hand." On the one hand, we did not have our typically large crowd of friends sharing matzo, matzo ball soup, gefilte fish and horseradish, brisket, and our flourless chocolate cake. On the other hand, because the pandemic closed the schools, our elder daughter was home from college, my husband and our younger daughter did not head off to campus/school early the next morning, and I was home all day to prepare food. A rare experience: we actually had our Seder on the traditional first night of Passover rather than waiting until the weekend when it would be convenient for our guests and for us.

That evening, just before we started the seder, we called my mother, who lives in a retirement community in Atlanta. Her apartment building was on complete lockdown after one of the residents tested positive for the coronavirus. But just after we hung up, my younger daughter suggested we call her back on FaceTime and have her be part of the Seder. So, we did that—we called her back on FaceTime and set the phone on a corner of the dining table so that she could see everyone.

Although it's possible we would have thought to do that under "normal" circumstances, I don't think that we would have. Shifting our lives into our houses for long periods of time, working from home, and having no places to congregate, we have moved much of our social lives—whether teaching, work meetings, or social gatherings—to Zoom or other online platforms.

We are now socializing online not only with people far away, but also with people who live nearby, thus changing how we think about what it means to socialize. The most mundane of activities like having a drink together is no longer possible. Thus, moving to an online version just to say hello means we are now thinking differently about how to connect with people.

CONCLUSION

Temple Israel in Memphis, Tennessee, is my "home" synagogue. I have been a member of the congregation since 1992; I had an adult bat mitzvah there in 1995; my husband and I were married there in 2000; and we had our younger daughter's baby naming with our rabbi in Memphis in 2004. I am tethered to that synagogue and was grateful when I could stream their services for the High Holidays.

Experiencing services in this way is certainly not as meaningful as being present in person, sitting in that beautiful sanctuary, looking around at familiar faces whom I have seen over so many years. But I was grateful nonetheless to be part of a service that has always moved me and to hear a sermon from rabbis who always make me think and feel deeply about my relationship to Judaism.

The social isolation from this pandemic, however, has pushed us to think differently about how to visit with people, how to socialize, and how to engage in religious ritual because now we must. The move to online social gathering is not even close to ideal, but it also opens a space for a possibility that did not exist previously—for family and friends to participate together in a ritual when even under normal circumstances they would not have been able to do so. But not being able to share a meal together will for me always be a marker of how impoverished the online ritual is.

What the pandemic revealed is that while staying alive is unbelievably significant, living a life of flourishing—a life that includes art, music, and social companionship; a life that is meaningful and lived in a meaningful way—is deeply important. I am not a frontline worker and I am grateful for their sacrifices in ways that I could never repay. My hope as a philosophy professor is to add to the dimension of life that nourishes the soul, that helps people understand why they would want to live and how they can create a life that is both meaningful and ethically responsive to others.

NOTES

1. Several paragraphs of this paper were originally published in Claire Katz, "Zooming into Passover," 21–23, in *Religion in Quarantine: The Future of Religion in a Post-Pandemic World*, ed. Heidi C. Campbell (College Station, TX: Digital Religion Publications, 2020), https://doi.org/10.21423/religioninquarantine; vailable electronically from https://hdl.handle.net/1969.1/188004.

I am grateful to Anna Gotlib for her helpful comments on earlier drafts of this chapter.

2. The original tweet by Lauren Morrill can be found here: https://twitter.com/laurenemorrill/status/819714138213642241?lang=en. It reads: "My biggest problem in these ACA debates? I don't know how to explain to you why you should care about other people," January 12, 2017, accessed online May 15, 2021.

On July 17, 2020, the website *Truth or Fiction* printed a response to the question, "Did Dr. Facui say, 'I don't know how to explain to you why you should care about other people'?" The site indicated that this was misattributed to Fauci. https://www.truthorfiction.com/did-dr-fauci-say-i-dont-know-how-to-explain-to-you-that-you-should-care-for-other-people/, accessed online May 15, 2021.

Georgia Public Broadcasting republished a piece first heard on *All Things Considered* confirming this misattribution: Rickey Bevington, "Macon Author's Words Wrongly Attributed to Dr. Anthony Fauci in Viral Posts," August 31, 2020, https://www.gpb.org/news/2020/08/31/macon-authors-words-wrongly-attributed-dr-anthony-fauci-in-viral-posts, accessed online May 15, 2021.

3. Kayla Chadwick, "I Don't Know How to Explain to You That You Should Care about Other People," *Huffington Post*, June 26, 2017, https://www.huffpost.com/entry/i-dont-know-how-to-explain-to-you-that-you-should_b_59519811e4b0f078efd98440, accessed online May 15, 2021.

4. Claire Elise Katz, *Levinas and the Crisis of Humanism* (Bloomington: Indiana University Press, 2013).

5. Blaise Pascal, *Thoughts*, section 5, Justice and the Reason of Effects, 295,

https://www.gutenberg.org/files/18269/18269-h/18269-h.htm, accessed online May 15, 2021.

6. Katz, *Levinas and the Crisis of Humanism*, 2.

7. Katz, *Levinas and the Crisis of Humanism*, 5

8. Katz, *Levinas and the Crisis of Humanism*, 5

9. Katz, *Levinas and the Crisis of Humanism* 5–6, emphasis added.

10. Kirsten Hall, "'Frederick": A Mouse with a Message," *Publishers Weekly*, July 28, 2020, https://www.publishersweekly.com/pw/by-topic/childrens/childrens-book-news/article/83970-frederick-a-mouse-with-a-message.html, accessed online March 14, 2021.

11. These next several paragraphs are from Katz, "Zooming into Passover," 21–23.

Chapter 11

Who Will I Be after All This Is Over?

Barrett Emerick

THE STRANGENESS OF LIMINALITY AND AUTOBIOGRAPHY

I don't do well with uncertainty.[1] I'm someone who wants to know where things stand in my friendships with others even at the risk of having awkward conversations. It's not that I feel insecure or doubt those relationships (though of course sometimes I do); it's that I want to know if I've made a misstep so I can work to correct it and be a better friend, or so that we can end the relationship, if that's what we need to do. One way or the other, I want to know (and am deeply uncomfortable not knowing) where things stand in my life. This has been a hard year.

I learned about "liminality" from philosopher Alison Reiheld when teaching her work on miscarriage in my undergraduate bioethics class. Reiheld describes liminality as "the betwixt and between-ness; something that is transitional, occupying a space between two poles, neither wholly one or the other."[2] She gives a number of examples of things, in addition to miscarriage, that can occupy such a liminal space: parenthood, procreation, even death (which can seem so final, so absolute, so . . . certain). My students, who had studied the concept in art classes, talked about standing in a doorway, neither in one room nor the other, between spaces in a way that defies full description and belies being totally pinned down. The deep strangeness of the spring 2020 semester includes the fact that I was lucky to have Reiheld visit my class via Skype, just one day before spring break. I've been teaching remotely, due to the COVID-19 pandemic, ever since. The first question in my lecture notes, in anticipation of her visit, was, “We’re in the beginning of an unfolding pandemic. Is this a liminal event?”

It is the strangeness of it all that continues to surprise me. Early on, it was the strangeness of following the news as the virus spread, spot after spot turning hot, knowing that it was coming and watching my government do so little to prepare. Then it was the strangeness of the virus itself: Because many people carried COVID-19 but were asymptomatic, and because many others had mild cases rather than severe, it was easy not to know if I had caught it or not. As I write this, I am not sick, and to my knowledge have not been sick, although there were several days where I felt strange or had a cough and wondered whether something worse was on the horizon. My partner and I are lucky (in so many ways) to have been able to mostly stay at home, to risk little exposure, to watch as the virus burned across the world. Not sick . . . not yet? Pre-sick? Alive and healthy; who knows for how long?

This chapter itself is a strange thing to write. It is certainly the most autobiographical thing I have ever published. It was inspired by a similar piece of autobiography in the *New York Times* by Gabrielle Hamilton, the owner of a restaurant in New York called Prune. Early in the pandemic, she had to close her restaurant, not knowing if it would reopen (and not knowing if there would be a place in the world for a restaurant like hers on the other side). Having been lucky to eat at Prune, I found her piece deeply moving and have thought of it many times as I grappled with the uncertainty of my own life and professional identity.[3]

This chapter is not only deeply personal but deals with the politics of higher education, specifically as it has played out at my own institution over the last couple of years via a process called “program prioritization.” The pandemic accelerated that process at many schools, either by making a college’s financial situation more precarious or by providing political cover to make cuts for other reasons. Those same patterns have played out in many workplaces beyond those in academia; it’s my hope that this piece might be helpful to others who are grappling with their own situations of uncertainty and precarity.

DISORIENTATION

The philosopher Ami Harbin calls disorienting events “temporally extended, major life experiences that make it difficult for individuals to know how to go on. They often involve feeling deeply out of place, unfamiliar, or not at home.”[4] She says that to be disoriented feels like “one loses one’s footing and is adrift in deep, unpredictable waters. In many such cases, it seems impossible that life will go on. Yet it does, and individuals can be carried along with it."[5]

Harbin's book *Disorientation and Moral Life* has been a salve for me throughout the pandemic. In articulating, analyzing, and unpacking "disorientation," it gave me an anchor to hold on to while the rest of my life felt so adrift. At least I could name what I was experiencing, and as is so often the case via the act of naming, come to be able to identify what was going on for me. "Real-life disorientations prompt individuals to morally and politically salient changes in action, and especially to new ways of relating to, caring for, acting with, and relying on other people, often apart from those individuals first deciding to do so. Crucially, disorientations can help us act even when we do not reorient."[6] Harbin's exploration of "resolve" is just as helpful as her exploration of "disorientation." As Harbin describes it, "resolve" has two meanings: On the one hand, when someone is in a position to "know what to do, how to do it, and have confidence, they can *resolve how to act* (in the sense of judging how to act)."[7] At the same time, in doing so they are thereby enabled to "*act with resolve* (in the sense of acting decisively, with determination, and confidence)."[8]

Liminality—the in-betweenness of one state or another, neither fully in the room nor fully outside the room—can sometimes be a profoundly disorienting experience. How can you resolve how to act if you are not fully in one space or the other? I take it liminality can also be experienced positively, where you are in both spaces at once; instead of neither one nor the other, it is instead both one and the other. If your social or professional role is ambiguous—what hat should I wear in giving this advice?—it can be difficult to know how to proceed, and so the advice you offer might therefore be tentative or hesitant. Of course, that's a good reason to communicate transparently about where you and the advice seeker both are coming from in having the conversation that you have. In that case, the liminal space is easily traversed; you can move through the doorway and into one room or the other rather than occupying a space in both.

Although Harbin's focus is on *moral* resolve—what is the morally right thing for me to do when I feel disoriented?—the resolve I have sought throughout the last year is personal. And I really mean that: I don't know who I will be, what *person* I will be, after the pandemic. Specifically, I don't know if my career will survive the pandemic, and so I don't know whether the person that I am will survive, either.

THE PROFESSIONAL IS PERSONAL (OR IT CAN BE)

I'm a philosophy professor, tenured at a small, public, teaching-intensive liberal arts college in 2017. Like so many schools, mine has struggled for years with declining enrollments and rising costs. Though we aren't as precarious as many, we are in real danger (facing what administrators have called an "existential threat"). Going into spring break in the middle of March 2020 was an exercise in liminality. The semester had started so well. For the first time in what felt like a long while, I was really excited, really up for teaching. That hopeful excitement was short-lived. In response to the "existential threat" of our declining enrollments, my college had begun a process of "program prioritization." Administrators and members of our board of trustees scratched their heads, confused as to why anyone would find such an effort demoralizing. The goal, after all, was simply to evaluate and rank academic programs on campus in terms of their importance to the future of the college. That type of rational ordering of means and ends was just good business; why all the fuss? Set aside the profound misunderstanding of what higher education is for, as well as the way program prioritization undermines our ability to satisfy our mission, and focus instead on what the term itself communicates: One program simply is more important than another, determined almost entirely by the extent to which it is profitable. Perplexed by my and other colleagues' resistance, administrators told us repeatedly that we shouldn't take it personally because they weren't, and it was not a reflection of whether they as individuals thought our disciplines were valuable but whether our disciplines would be a good draw for high school students making the choice where to lay down a deposit (setting aside the obvious, which is that most high school students have no idea what philosophy even is).

"Don't take it personally." What an absurd thing to say—to offer as consolation to someone whose personal identity is so utterly bound up with, so thoroughly constituted by, your professional identity—as they engage in a process whose sole purpose is to prioritize some areas of teaching and research over yours. What is more personal than telling someone that their identity, once relatively stable and fixed, is now itself liminal? It feels like being slowly thrown away, of being rendered obsolete while you still haunt the campus—no longer a full member of the community and contributor to the future of the institution but still in some ways a part of things, occupying the same roles that you once did.

I mean it when I say that I'm not sure I will survive the pandemic. At this point, I just *am* a philosopher. I don't mean here to suggest that I was born a philosopher (though I can look back on my early childhood and find the foundations of my philosophical inclinations sitting there so obviously that this identity seems a forgone conclusion). Instead, I have worked very hard to become a philosopher, starting in 2002, when I decided at the end of college that this was who I wanted to be and what I wanted to do. Since that day, all my professional effort has pointed me down this road. It is, for me, an orientation: a way of approaching the world, relationships, current events, and popular culture. Philosophers are (for better or worse) my people: We speak the same language, ears perking up when certain kinds of claims are made, terms used, examples given. We not only share similar types of work and working conditions, we share the same pool of knowledge and set of conceptual resources to make sense of the world. Many of them feel like my kin.

I don't mean to suggest that all philosophers are the same. We are infamous for being exclusive to anyone who doesn't look like me (a white man), although I have hope about ways in which the demographics of the discipline are becoming more diverse due to the tireless efforts of many to remove barriers of entry and make it less hostile. Philosophers are also notorious for our infighting, argumentative brutality, arrogance, and for refusing to leave our place at the very top of the ivory tower, so far from the ground that we talk about issues that matter to actual human beings as if they are mere puzzles to be solved. But not all philosophers are like this, and increasingly I find hope also in the nonideal turn, living much more happily down on the ground, engaging with the experience and insights that come from living real lives, taking seriously the messiness and contingency of the real world, theorizing not from nowhere but from here and now, with actual history and the legacies of violence, oppression, and domination setting the stage for whatever conclusions we reach.

I was not always this kind of philosopher. I started out happy to take a much more idealized stance, to play with thought experiments involving violence and death like the now-famous trolley case and debate them with other grad students late into the night. I'm lucky to have studied under some of the philosophers who are responsible for helping to bring about the "nonideal turn"—who specialized in philosophical methodology and forced (and are forcing) the rest of the discipline into a reckoning with our own abstraction, detachment, and the privilege that enables both. Today, as I meet and connect with philosophers on social media and at conferences, I am happy to say that so many brilliant colleagues and friends are doing work from the ground and not from the clouds, turning the tools of philosophy to good use to help us better understand the world, what it means to be a person, and what it means to matter.

My research focus has been to explore agents' inner lives, both as sites where profound injury and injustice play out and as sites of repair and resistance. That has meant, among other things, thinking about what emotions are, what they can do for us, when they are morally appropriate, and what they can tell us about the world. In perhaps my favorite piece of philosophy, my teacher Alison Jaggar argues that "Only when we reflect on our initially puzzling irritability, revulsion, anger or fear may we bring to consciousness our 'gut-level' awareness that we are in a situation of coercion, cruelty, injustice, or danger."[9] Here Jaggar is describing what she calls "outlaw emotions" (those emotions that are unconventional or run counter to dominant ideologies or social imaginaries).[10] But emotions can be revelatory more generally, and by paying attention to how we feel we can learn things about our circumstances, the relationships in which we participate, or the way we are being treated. That's not to say that our emotions always track the world perfectly or accurately—as Jaggar says, "Although our emotions are epistemologically indispensable, they are not epistemologically indisputable."[11] Instead, it is to say that our emotional responses can be one method of learning new things and justifying our beliefs.[12] In analyzing bitterness (an emotion to which I will return), Lynne McFall claims that feeling bitter can serve as a method of "bearing witness" or of "truth-telling."[13] The feeling itself, as well as its expression, is a type of testimony to the circumstances in which it is felt, or of the treatment the one who feels it has suffered. "And where the truth is harsh, and of human origin, and avoidable, bitterness is a form of moral accounting, of naming the losses, that we can condone both in ourselves and others."[14] I take it that paying careful attention to our emotional responses can be one method of grappling with disorientation and achieving some resolve. One origin of disorientation is not knowing how you're feeling or experiencing feelings that are in conflict. On the other hand, by identifying those feelings and their causes, you might then be able to choose how to act and to do so with confidence.

It's my aim in this (most personal) chapter to listen to my own emotional life and learn from it what I can about the deeply disorienting experience of the last year. It is also my aim to engage in the moral accounting McFall describes, to articulate and name some of the losses (and the wrongs) that program prioritization has wrought at my school (and that it has and will inflict at schools, both large and small, across the United States). Specifically, when I pay attention to how I'm feeling (and how I have been feeling since program prioritization began) and try to make sense of my emotions and give them space to testify to the nature of my circumstances, it becomes clear that it is, among other things, anticipatory grief that I am feeling, for a death on my life's horizon.

GRIEF

There are different types of death. As Thomas Nagel argues in his classic essay, physical death is bad because it deprives someone of all that is good—it is an evil of deprivation of the goods of life: being able to experience beauty, to desire things and have those desires satisfied, to do things, to think, believe, and care about things, to be in relationship with and to care about (and to be cared for by) others. "The trouble is that life familiarizes us with the goods of which death deprives us. . . . Having been gratuitously introduced to the world by a collection of natural, historical, and social accidents, he [*sic*] finds himself [*sic*] the subject of a *life*, with an indeterminate and not essentially limited future."[15] Physical death would end the opportunity for me to do all of those things; its finality (once it is final) will mean being deprived of all of those goods that my physical life brings with it. If my life as a philosopher ends, I will still be able to do so many of those things, and I do not for a second mean to diminish the permanent and thoroughgoing loss so many people have suffered from COVID-19. But it is a death nonetheless—a death of who I have been for almost all my adult life—and one that seems more imminent by the day.

Some friends have told me, in a well-intentioned effort to provide comfort, that I'll always be a philosopher, even if I leave academia. That might be true for some people, but for me, part of being a philosopher is the doing of philosophy—reading and writing, presenting work and commenting on the work of others, planning to do all those things and letting ideas simmer in the background while I'm doing chores or awake at 2:00 a.m.—and of course teaching. If I have to leave academia, I will leave all (or almost all) of those things behind. While I will likely still retain the philosophical orientation I've had since I was little, and while I'll hold on to the concepts and method I've acquired throughout my professional training, I won't be a philosopher anymore. If I'm not doing philosophy in a robust way, it won't make sense to me to think of myself as a philosopher. And, as Nagel argued, having been acquainted with the goods of that life, I now face the bad of being deprived of them as I anticipate the untimely death of that part of who I am.

And so I realized at some point in the last year as program prioritization ramped up at my school and as it concluded its work at other schools (as friends and colleagues started to lose their jobs or be forced into early retirement) that I was grieving for a life cut short, deprived of the goods that would have accompanied its continuance. *I'm not ready to go*: In many ways I feel like I've just gotten started, that my research agenda has only recently gelled into a unified whole. I felt fortunate to secure a good job right out of graduate school. My new colleagues encouraged me to take my time in publishing and focus on finding my feet in the classroom, at the school, and in the discipline. That was well-intentioned advice with which I agree: The arms race to publish makes the discipline worse overall. Philosophy often needs to simmer for years before it is ready to serve, and there is too much out there written (understandably) too quickly by people needing to build their CVs. Even though I knew that I would need to publish more if I wanted to be able to move on to another college, I was happy where I was and decided to try to put down roots. I wanted to be a part of an institution that invested deeply in its students, that had a sense of identity and shared purpose, that valued the liberal arts and the transformative work that can be done in a small classroom. I knew that it would be hard to leave the longer I stayed but thought that tenure—what I believed to be a lifetime appointment—at such an institution would be worth working to achieve. That security, that permanence of my own identity as bound up with that particular place, was worth the sacrifice of mobility. After all, I love teaching first and best, but also believed I could still be a part of the larger philosophical community and that I would have enough time each summer to write. I never aspired to be a rock star, but I did want my work to matter. I wanted my voice to join the chorus of others in the literature that have meant so much to me and to my students, in the hopes that it would be of use.

I still want that—I still hope for it. But I no longer know whether that desire is achievable, whether that hope can be realized. Some days it feels certain that my career is ending; others, I can't get my head around that possibility, can't conceive of who I would be if not a philosopher. My professional identity—and whether it is something to grieve—has itself become liminal. Logging into my Zoom classroom to meet with my students has become surreal, disorienting, uncertain. Will I be at the college next year to supervise their senior theses? If they choose to hold off on taking a class with me until next spring when it better fits with their course needs, will I be around to teach it? Of course, life is fragile, and I know that such uncertainty is always on the scene, in the background of all such conversations. But this feels like an active uncertainty, not lurking in the background but in the middle of the room, burning up all the oxygen it can.

How much of this should I share with my students? A favorite professor in graduate school taught me much of what I know about teaching. One day, she said what should have been obvious but that I think it can sometimes be easy to forget: Our students are not our therapists. At the same time, I think it's good to be recognizable to them as a whole, complete person and to treat them as they are: like adults capable of responding reasonably and appropriately to hard news. We also owe them that transparency and honesty: They deserve to know what's going on at their school, what looms on the horizon for their major, or whether they'll have the opportunity to take a class next year or not. This, again, is liminal—are we a major or not? Is this area of study one that is valued or not? The question of personal-professional identity I have been grappling with and the uncertainty of whether it is one thing or the other, alive or dead, ongoing or over, is thereby translated over to our major and the college more generally. Are we a liberal arts college or not? Our president has reassured us that we will always be a liberal arts college—just a liberal arts college for the twenty-first century. Cold comfort.

So yes, I have been grieving. The professional is personal—or it is for me—and who I am as a person has been imperiled by many threats. Already meager enrollments are predicted to be made worse by a demographic "cliff" in 2026 in which the number of eighteen-year-olds in the United States will steeply decline. Small colleges have already started to close across the country; many more will follow in their wake, and many others will use those facts as justification to dramatically remake curricular offerings and institutional identities. COVID-19 has accelerated those cuts and closures, often serving as an excuse to justify them.[16] Boards of trustees across the country, mostly populated by people who have no experience in higher education, will decide what should and should not be taught, which disciplines are valuable and high priority and which are merely fluff, fat that can be cut, a distraction from the real work of preparing students to enter the workforce. In making those decisions, they will fail to pay attention to the quantitative data (which they will always claim to want) that say that real job preparedness is in fact served by a true liberal arts education, that the arts and humanities actually serve not only that goal but at the same time also the goal of helping students to become more complete people, better able to live meaningful and responsible lives, to contribute to the world—and, yes, to be accomplished professionals.

My grief is not just for the death of my own professional identity, but for the death of higher education in the United States. Of course, philosophy and other "low-priority" disciplines will still be taught at the Ivies and the elite (and well-heeled) liberal arts colleges. It is ironic that in an age where we talk constantly about diversity, equity, and inclusion in higher education and in corporate America, one of the great goods of life—the opportunity to formally study such disciplines—will be available only to the elite or the wealthy. I hope that I'm wrong; this near future is itself uncertain and things might go a different way. But after two years of steeping in it, that alternative is hard to imagine.

ANGER AND BITTERNESS

So far, I've been describing the way that paying attention to my grief has been both clarifying and disorienting throughout program prioritization for which

COVID-19 has been an accelerant. It has helped me to make sense of my situation: What I have been doing is grieving the end of a life. It is also disorienting: Is this life actually ending? What am I to do now? These are questions that so many people have asked themselves throughout the pandemic as their careers have been destroyed, their savings drained, their relationships strained or severed.

Grief is not the only emotion that has been simultaneously clarifying and disorienting. While grief has hummed along in the background, it has often been punctuated with bouts of intense anger (the moral emotion I've thought about the most in my work). The philosopher P. F. Strawson tells us in his canonical "Freedom and Resentment" that though we might feel anger *that* some bad state of affairs obtains (we might feel angry that a lightning bolt burned down our house) we feel angry *with* moral agents (with people), whom we can hold responsible for their wrongful actions.[17] Anger, like grief, can be epistemically valuable—it can help us to learn new things about the world. Anger with the arsonist reflects the judgement that they are a person rather than a naturally occurring event. It makes the claim that they could have done otherwise and ought to have done so. And it is predicated on the judgement that the owner of the house they destroyed is a person themself who deserved to be treated differently, with respect.

Perhaps it is gratuitous to unpack the ways in which I have felt angry this past year. Again, throughout COVID-19 there have been uncountably many horrors, massive amounts of avoidable suffering, all more significant and profound than the possible loss of my career and professional identity. To say that anger expresses the moral judgement that an action was wrongful is not to say that the absence of anger entails the absence of that judgement. As Strawson tells us, resentment is a *personal* reactive attitude; the moral anger I experience is born from the wrongs that I or my loved ones experience or that threaten us. Certainly, I can be angry (and am often angry) about wrongs that I have not personally suffered, but those that affect me directly are felt more acutely, grounded in self-defense or the defense of those loved ones with whom my self is bound up.

It has been a struggle, this year, to grapple with my anger. It comes in waves and is at times scalding and destructive. My anger has been directed at various members of my college for, among other things, a stunning lack of vision and sense of shared identity, for the willingness to remain oblivious to what the outcomes of program prioritization would be, for the willingness to comply with whatever directives they were given, or for being too self-interested to do otherwise. I've been angry with a system that invests the board of trustees with this type of oversight and decision-making power and with board members themselves for manifesting the special type of hubris that is born from being rich in a society that equates wealth with expertise and competence. And it has been directed toward myself: I should have written more; I should have invested more in building my CV and advancing farther and faster in my career; I should have been more focused and specialized in my research. And, more than anything, I am angry at myself for my naivete; I trusted that the college I had joined would keep its promises, that if I was a good teacher and a good scholar I would be valued, and that tenure would mean I could take my time in becoming the scholar I *still* aspire to be. What a fool I have been, all these long years.

I had understood tenure to mean lifetime employment for those who earned it, and that as long as the college exists and tenured faculty don't commit acts of "moral turpitude," they would have a job. When it became clear in the fall of 2020 that faculty would in fact be fired, I made the point to colleagues that there was now a two-tiered tenure system at the college; those faculty in large majors that are valued as being practical choices for students or that attract students to the college had tenure as I had understood it, while those of us in small programs or with supposedly impractical disciplines had no such assurance. After I voiced this double-standard, one colleague in my department pointed out that of course that had always been the case and that small majors like ours have always been vulnerable to cuts in light of politics or financial exigency (or the former under the cover of the latter). That I saw immediately that he was right was no balm for the outrageousness of it all and no salve for the burns the self-directed anger inflicted for my own folly in ever thinking otherwise.

As time has passed, some of the anger has burned out and left bitterness behind. McFall analyzes bitterness as being born from the disappointment of one's important and legitimate hopes in the absence of excusing conditions.[18] That last bit is important: So much of the badness of program prioritization has been avoidable, inexcusable, culpable. If the college had sought, from the beginning, to meaningfully include the faculty as a whole (not to mention staff, students, and alumni) in the process, not only would the end result be different and less destructive, but it would be more legitimate. If we had collectively been given the opportunity to face the real existential threat of declining enrollments together, as a community, we could have worked to avoid a second existential threat that has loomed in the background throughout the entire process: no longer being the same institution (or same type of institution) that we once were. Only time will tell who the institution will become, though it seems very likely to me that that second type of existential threat will be actualized in horrific, excruciating slowness over the next decade, as additional programs are eliminated and faculty who are not outright fired or forced to retire will be left to (as one administrator put it) "wither on the vine." Liminality is endemic to that process: not what we were, not what we will be; the “betwixt and betweenness” of the slow death of a once great institution.

HOPE

Like many others, I have a complicated relationship with hope. On one hand, it seems easily dashed or misplaced; worse, it serves as an excuse for inaction or “bad faith” in which I hope that someone else will sweep in and save the day, rescuing me from my circumstances and delivering me to better things. Jean-Paul Sartre tells us that “The genius of Proust is the totality of the works of Proust. . . . Why would we attribute to Racine the capacity to write yet another tragedy when that is precisely what he did not write?”[19] Sartre, not one to mince words, goes on to say, “No doubt this thought may seem comfortless to one who has not made a success of his [*sic*] life. On the other hand, it puts everyone in a position to understand that reality alone is reliable; that dreams, expectations, and hopes serve to define a man [*sic*] only as deceptive dreams and abortive hopes, expectations unfulfilled; that is to say, they define him [*sic*] negatively, not positively.”[20] I take Sartre to be arguing that all that we are is what we undertake and accomplish. To look at my life and say, “I could have been a great philosopher but my time was cut short” is to pass the buck to others and deny that I could have done more, could have made more of the (already abundant) opportunities that I had, and that I failed to take responsibility for not being who I wanted or for making of my life all that I wanted it to be.

On the other hand, it seems that hope is essential to agency, and that to live as a person (in perhaps exactly the authentic way Sartre describes) requires that I invest in the idea that my will could go somewhere, do something, that my effort could find purchase and have the intended effect.[21] Perhaps these two views are reconciled in the work of Rebecca Solnit, who says, in writing about the relationship between hope and activism, that the “future is dark”—not in the sense of being bad, but of being unknown. Furthermore, she argues that that lack of certainty—that darkness and indeterminacy—is good because it leaves open exactly the space for agential effort to find purchase. Despair, on the other hand, “presumes it knows what will happen next” and in that way lets the cynic off the hook for having to try. “If everything is doomed, then nothing is required.”[22]

As I read Solnit, it is a type of self-indulgence to let myself be miserable. I have needed to work through and try to achieve some understanding of what has happened and where I am in my life’s story so that I can find a way forward despite lacking the resolve to act that disorientation has compromised. This has been incredibly hard, and the future remains dark. I don’t know whether who I have been will survive for much longer, but some version of me will. And after all, the world is much bigger than my silly little life. Solnit says,

> The future is bigger than our imaginations. It is unimaginable, and then it comes anyway. To meet it we need to keep going, to walk past what we can imagine. We need to be unstoppable. And here's what it takes: you don't stop walking to congratulate yourself; you don't stop walking to wallow in despair; you don't stop because your own life got too comfortable or too rough; you don't stop because you won; you don't stop because you lost. There's more to win, more to lose, others who need you.
>
> You don't stop walking because there is no way forward. Of course there is no way. You walk the path into being, you make the way, and if you do it well, others can follow the route. You look backward to grasp the long history you're moving forward from, the paths others have made, the road you came in on. You look forward to possibility. That's what we mean by hope, and you look past it into the impossible and that doesn't stop you either. But mostly you just walk, right foot, left foot, right food, left foot. That's what makes you unstoppable.[23]

CONCLUSION

One of the friends who was kind enough to read this chapter for me as I was revising it commented that she liked the previous section on hope but that it didn't seem like my heart was really in it. I think she's probably right; though I deeply value Solnit's insight and have relied on her words many times in the past, it's hard right now to take much comfort in them. Perhaps my hope is aspirational, or it is meta-hope—hope that I will one day hope. I remember a time where I believed in that kind of hope—not Pollyanna hope, not the bad faith of hoping someone will save me from my situation, but the authentic hope of taking one small step forward at a time, trusting in myself and those on whom I rely, and believing that I can make a way forward, even if right now that way is unknown to me. By choosing to include the section on hope, I am trusting not just others who believe in me now but my past self who thought that orientation valuable and appropriate.

And, regardless, you can't write something like this and just have it end with despair. People are generally uncomfortable with the negative feelings of others. McFall begins her discussion of bitterness by noting that "'You're so bitter' is condemnation, never praise,"[24] and that bitter people are rarely thought to be good dinner guests.[25] I would extend her insight to include the other challenging feelings I've explored throughout. Anger can feel dangerous; grief, painful. Disorientation, and the liminality from which it often emerges, is unattractive. As deeply social beings, humans must constantly respond (one way or the other) to the emotional lives of others; the expression of emotion calls out to us, hoping for recognition, empathy, solidarity, or support.[26] When those emotions are unpleasant, uncertain, unhappy, or messy it can be hard to respond, hard to know how to empathize, hard to not commit what Jean Harvey calls "moral abandonment" in which you leave the other to suffer alone.[27]

I am fortunate to have had many friends and family who love me and have not abandoned me throughout this experience. It is notable, though, that my grief, anger, and bitterness have more easily secured uptake with others in my life than has the experience of disorientation. It's just hard to know what to do with disorientation, both in our own lives and in the lives of those whom we love. Culturally, we value resolve, clarity of intention, and statements of purpose and vision. To be caught in the in-between space where such clarity is impossible and such resolve cannot thrive is, by its nature, a challenge to moral solidarity. It's often good practice just to sit with someone who is grieving or in pain rather than trying to fix it or repair the harm. How do you sit with someone who doesn't know where they are, who is "betwixt and between" being one way or another? How do you support someone and tell them you know they'll make it through the dark woods when their disorientation is so profound as to have left them with no sense of the way forward? One reason why Harbin's work is so valuable is because it helps to put not just grappling with our own disorientation but supporting others who are disoriented on our agenda; part of being in moral solidarity with others involves meeting them where they are, even when they don't know where that is. It also encourages us to be ok with disorientation itself, and to know that we can continue to act and find a way forward, even absent the certainty or resolve we often crave. Even if they don't know who they are or who they will be. Even if they doubt that who they are now will survive.

BIBLIOGRAPHY

Bader, Eleanor J. "Colleges Are Using COVID as a Pretext to Make Draconian Cuts to the Humanities." *Truthout*, March 28, 2021. https://truthout.org/articles/colleges-are-using-covid-as-a-pretext-to-make-draconian-cuts-to-the-humanities/.

Bell, MacAlester. "A Woman's Scorn: Toward a Feminist Defense of Contempt as a Moral Emotion," *Hypatia* 20, no. 4 (2005): 80–93.

Hamilton, Gabrielle. "My Restaurant Was My Life for 20 Years. Does the World Need It Anymore?" *New York Times*, April 23, 2020. https://www.nytimes.com/2020/04/23/magazine/closing-prune-restaurant-covid.html.

Harbin, Ami. *Disorientation and Moral Life*. New York: Oxford University Press, 2016.

Harvey, Jean. "Moral Solidarity and Empathetic Understanding: The Moral Value and Scope of the Relationship." *Journal of Social Philosophy* 38, no. 1 (2007): 22–37.

Jaggar, Alison M. "Love and Knowledge: Emotion in Feminist Epistemology," 378–91. In *Just Methods: An Interdisciplinary Feminist Reader*, ed. Alison M. Jaggar. New York: Taylor and Francis, 2014.

Lindemann, Hilde. *Holding and Letting Go: The Social Practice of Personal Identities*. New York: Oxford University Press, 2014.

McFall, Lynne. "What's Wrong with Bitterness?" 146–60. In *Feminist Ethics*, ed. Claudia Card. Lawrence: University Press of Kansas, 1991.

McGeer, Victoria. "The Art of Good Hope." *Annals of the American Academy of Political and Social Science* 592 (March 2004): 100–27.

Nagel, Thomas. "Death," *Nous* 4, no. 1 (1970): 73–80.

Reiheld, Alison. "'The Event That Was Nothing': Miscarriage as a Liminal Event." *Journal of Social Philosophy* 46, no. 1 (2015): 9–26.

Sartre, Jean-Paul. "Existentialism Is a Humanism," 345–69. In *Existentialism from Dostoevsky to Sartre*, ed. Walter Kaufman. New York: Penguin, 1975.

Solnit, Rebecca. "What Comes after Hope." *TomDispatch*, May 19, 2013. https://tomdispatch.com/rebecca-solnit-what-comes-after-hope/.

Stockdale, Katie. "Social and Political Dimensions of Hope." *Journal of Social Philosophy* 50, no. 1 (2019): 28–44.

Strawson, P. F. "Freedom and Resentment," 1–28. In *Freedom and Resentment and Other Essays*. New York: Routledge, 1974.

NOTES

1. I am very grateful to Shannon Dea, Jane Dryden, Anna Gotlib, Ami Harbin, Alice MacLachlan, Kate Norlock, Alison Reiheld, Kevin Timpe, and Audrey Yap for their invaluable insight, feedback, and support in writing this chapter.

2. Alison Reiheld, "'The Event That Was Nothing': Miscarriage as a Liminal Event," *Journal of Social Philosophy* 46, no. 1 (2015): 10.

3. Gabrielle Hamilton, "My Restaurant Was My Life for 20 Years. Does the World Need It Anymore?" *New York Times*, April 23, 2020, https: //www.nytimes.com/2020/04/23/magazine/closing-prune-restaurant-covid.html

4. Ami Harbin, *Disorientation and Moral Life* (New York: Oxford University Press, 2016), 2.

5. Harbin, *Disorientation and Moral Life*, 3.

6. Harbin, *Disorientation and Moral Life*, 34.

7. Harbin, *Disorientation and Moral Life*, 41.

8. Harbin, *Disorientation and Moral Life*, 41.

9. Alison M. Jaggar, "Love and Knowledge: Emotion in Feminist Epistemology," in *Just Methods: An Interdisciplinary Feminist Reader*, ed. Alison M. Jaggar (New York: Taylor and Francis, 2014), 387.

10. Jaggar, "Love and Knowledge," 387.

11. Jaggar, "Love and Knowledge," 389.

12. I take this to be another important way that the "nonideal turn" has played out in philosophy and in popular culture more generally. Today, my students are much more friendly to the idea that reason and emotion can happily work together than they were even ten years ago. For a helpful discussion of the epistemic value of emotion, see MacAlester Bell, "A Woman's Scorn: Toward a Feminist Defense of Contempt as a Moral Emotion," *Hypatia* 20, no. 4 (2005): 80–93.

13. Lynne McFall, "What's Wrong with Bitterness?" in *Feminist Ethics*, ed. Claudia Card (Lawrence: University Press of Kansas, 1991), 155.

14. McFall, "What's Wrong with Bitterness?" 156.

15. Thomas Nagel, "Death," *Nous* 4, no. 1 (1970): 80.

16. Eleanor J. Bader, "Colleges Are Using COVID as a Pretext to Make Draconian Cuts to the Humanities." *Truthout*, March 28, 2021, https://truthout.org/articles/colleges-are-using-covid-as-a-pretext-to-make-draconian-cuts-to-the-humanities/.

17. P. F. Strawson, "Freedom and Resentment," 1–28, in *Freedom and Resentment and Other Essays* (New York: Routledge, 1974).

18. McFall, "What's Wrong with Bitterness?" 150.

19. Jean-Paul Sartre, "Existentialism Is a Humanism," in *Existentialism from Dostoevsky to Sartre*, ed. Walter Kaufman (New York: Penguin, 1975_, 359.

20. Sartre, "Existentialism Is a Humanism," 359.

21. For more on the relationship between agency and hope see Victoria McGeer, "The Art of Good Hope," *Annals of the American Academy of Political and Social Science* 592 (March 2004): 100–27; and Katie Stockdale, "Social and Political Dimensions of Hope," *Journal of Social Philosophy* 50, no. 1 (2019): 28–44.

22. Rebecca Solnit, "What Comes after Hope," *TomDispatch*, May 19, 2013, https://tomdispatch.com/rebecca-solnit-what-comes-after-hope/.

23. Solnit, "What Comes after Hope."

24. McFall, "What's Wrong with Bitterness?" 146.

25. McFall, "What's Wrong with Bitterness?" 157.

26. Hilde Lindemann argues that personhood consists in the expression of our inner lives, recognition of that expression by others, and their subsequent response. Hilde Lindemann, *Holding and Letting Go: The Social Practice of Personal Identities* (New York: Oxford University Press, 2014).

27. Jean Harvey, "Moral Solidarity and Empathetic Understanding: The Moral Value and Scope of the Relationship," *Journal of Social Philosophy* 38, no. 1 (2007): 22–37.

Chapter 12

The COVID-19 Guidebook for Living in an Alternate Universe

Eyja M. Brynjarsdóttir

About thirty years ago, my address changed even though I did not move. A change in the planning of my hometown had the effect that a new street name was created for a part of my street, and my address was moved from the old street name to the new one with no effort on my behalf. This felt slightly strange but affected my life very little, except I had to fill out forms for change of address in a few places. The changes experienced in the first few weeks of the COVID-19 pandemic shared features of this experience, yet the experience was much more powerful. It was similar in the sense that it involved a move while staying still, but instead of a geographical move or a change of address, it involved a move to an alternate universe. Of course, I was by no means alone in this move; a great number of people had similar experiences, many of which, however, differed from mine to various degrees.

The COVID-19 pandemic has caused many of us to feel as if the whole world has shifted, even though we are more or less staying inside our very familiar homes. We have had to acquire all kinds of new knowledge very fast, from opinions on things we never thought about before, to worries about things we never even considered before. This has been accompanied by a feeling of surreality: While many of us have been stuck inside the same home, it has been moved to a different world. In our past, we have read books, watched movies and TV shows, and even played board games with dystopic storylines involving plagues, lockdown situations, people in isolation, and various other imminent threats and worldwide emergencies. We were suddenly pulled into the middle of such a storyline and forced to become participants in an alternate universe fantasy. The focus of this chapter is on the effects of this participation on the development and perception of the self. While great numbers of people have suffered enormous hardships due to the pandemic, and this is something that requires both acknowledgment and remediating action, the attention here is not on the resulting pain and suffering but on the world-altering effects of this move between worlds for all of us, even those of us lucky enough to have escaped with minimal harm. We suddenly find ourselves living in a viral outbreak movie. Which roles are we playing?

MOVING

Expect the move to be sudden. A move to an alternate universe happens without warning, and you will not realize until after the fact what has happened. Something makes the whole world shift, and you are taken elsewhere in spite of staying put. In some cases, you are to spend a great deal, or even all, of your time in your home. Others, however, may spend less time than usual at home, working under increased duress and facing increased risks at work.

Expect confusion at various points. A few weeks in, you will keep thinking back to how life was only a few weeks ago and contrast it with the now. You will be struck with a feeling of unreality, and you will wonder whether you are dreaming. You are not dreaming.

You will unexpectedly learn about things you never thought would ever interest you, and even become obsessed with some of them. Perhaps you will take a sudden interest in reading articles on the ideal method for handwashing, various aspects of what viruses are and what they do, possible transmission methods of viruses, the pros and cons of mask use and glove use, and the effects of social distancing on viral transmission. You will then have arguments with other people about all of these things. You will learn about something called "epidemiology," and with it, about the exponential spread of viral diseases, their social effects, and how outbreaks that are only lethal for a small proportion of the population can still have disastrous effects and overflow the healthcare system. You will keep track of how many urgent care beds there are in hospitals in your area as well as the number of functioning respirators. The most unlikely of your acquaintances will now have strong opinions on things you never thought they knew anything about, such as how to calculate and evaluate optimal epidemiological methods for containing viral spread. You will learn countless new terms.

Expect to learn about the impacts of a plague that you had never considered. Unemployment and loss of income. Uncertainty about the future. Overworked healthcare professionals under extreme pressure. Cutting of various highly important services for children, the elderly, and people with disabilities. What happens when the schools close and there is no tourism?

What jobs can be performed from home? What do you need to learn in order to work from home? How do parents solve the problem of working full-time from home while taking care of children whose education is now virtual? What happens when those suffering domestic abuse have to spend weeks on end in isolation in their homes with their abusers? What are the effects on a society when certain groups of people are more susceptible than others to severe and even lethal effects of a viral disease and require protection in isolation from the rest of us? How do various people respond to the threat of a plague? How do *you* respond? Will you be in the cautious or the reckless group? Are you in one of the especially vulnerable groups? Do you have friends or family members belonging to a risk group, or do you feel that you and yours are safe? What are your opinions on the best ways to respond to the various problems that arise and that you knew very little about only a few weeks earlier?

Gradually, you may come to realize that while there are all sorts of new issues in your own environment, those in other environments, and in other parts of the world, may be considerably different, and in some cases more severe. This can also be true of people in your own vicinity, even your next-door neighbors. They may be enduring effects of the pandemic that are very different from those you have felt. This may result in very different points of view when it comes to prioritizing needs and evaluating different possible actions.

Expect to discover new sides of yourself, as well as the possibility that things almost never turn out the way you expect them to. For example, if your area is under lockdown, you may in the beginning form plans for various home improvement projects, bread baking, nice family time, and, in general, for working on your domestic virtues. Do expect most of these plans to fail. Expect to get really frustrated with yourself at times. But you might also discover, as you and your family members burst into song and silly dance moves, that you have spent too much time in isolation.

SETTLING

I have suffered from chronic migraines for most of my life, ever since I was a child, impacting my lifestyle and quality of life in various negative ways. I certainly do not like getting a headache, and I usually feel disappointed when I get one yet again. During some periods in my life, I have managed to get rid of the migraines for a while, for a few weeks or even months. When that happened, I felt enormous relief and liberation. Yet there is some part of me that also begins to miss the old pain in my head. When I finally get a headache,

I sense a feeling of comfort and familiarity, even though it would not make sense to say that I am happy about it.

After some months of confusion and a state of unreality, you, too, may begin to get accustomed to your new circumstances, much to your surprise. It is even possible that you begin to feel so well-adjusted that you dread the return to the old "normal." You may think to yourself: "Is it really necessary to go to work at a workplace every day, meet people in person, and walk around without a face mask?" This may happen even if you face various difficulties while juggling family life and work at home, feel lonely without the encounters with others—not to mention worries about your health and that of others or about those who have it much worse than you. To some degree, perhaps we have a tendency to get accustomed to any circumstance, even though we never wished for it and would consider it far from ideal, and even if it causes discomfort and pain. So much mental energy has been spent learning about life in the "new normal" that we begin to forget how things were done before, and thus feel insecure about returning to that kind of life.

When the situation is new, we are strongly aware of the sense of novelty and surreality. Gradually, this feeling may begin to fade away and the alternate universe becomes the norm. Of course, we all have previous experiences of adjustment, of something new becoming normal and then even old, such as when shiny new shoes gradually become familiar and worn-out. But the level of adjustment needed in this situation is greater than previously experienced by most of us. Moving to a new place can, of course, involve great changes and require many adjustments, but in this particular situation, the old "place" does not seem to exist anymore, at least not for the time being. Homes can also be ruined by wars or natural disasters. The situation most of us experience due to the pandemic does for most of us not involve the trauma experienced by those displaced through terrible, tragic events, but we are still likely to feel disoriented and confused.

POINTS OF REFERENCE

A move between worlds will also change our points of reference, affecting the meaning of words and also our means of accessing and thinking about various other things. In his papers "Meaning and Reference"[1] and "The Meaning of Meaning,"[2] the philosopher Hilary Putnam presented his highly influential Twin Earth argument for a theory called semantic externalism. According to semantic externalism, the meaning of the words we use is not solely determined by the thoughts inside our heads, or what we *intend* for the words to mean, but also by various states of affairs in the world surrounding us. For example, when I use the word "horse," I have an idea about what that word represents and I have an intention to use this word about a certain kind of animal corresponding to that idea. However, I could have misunderstood and have the wrong idea about what horses are like. In that case, the meaning of the word I am using would not be corresponding to the idea inside my head. The external factors determining or affecting the meaning of words can be social, but they can also be facts about the natural world. This view has been famously summarized as "'meanings' just ain't in the head."

Now, getting back to Putnam's Twin Earth argument: The idea was that we should imagine a place, Twin Earth, that is identical to our Earth in every way except that the substance there called "water," that is found in raindrops and rivers, that most living beings require for their survival, and so on, does not have the chemical composition H_2O, but XYZ. We are then to imagine a person, Oscar, in our world, and his counterpart, Twin-Oscar, on Twin Earth. They are in every respect the same, but when our Oscar uses the word "water," he is referring to the substance H_2O, and when Twin-Oscar utters "water," he is referring to XYZ. Putnam's point is that the meaning of a term is determined not only by the speakers' mental states, but also by the conditions of their surroundings. We can then think of "our" Oscar being transferred to Twin Earth. While there, he may point to a clear liquid in a glass, that others nearby are calling "water," and say, "This is water." In that case, Oscar is speaking falsely, because as he is from Earth, he is actually stating (and thinking) that there is H_2O in the glass, while what is actually in the glass is XYZ.[3]

Of course, Putnam's Twin Earth case is not perfectly analogous with the transport between worlds that I have been describing. Our new alternate universe is *not* indistinguishable from the regular old one; after all, the feeling of an alternate universe is due to all those sudden changes that we have actually experienced. And Putnam's argument concerns how the meaning of words is determined, which is not what I am about to discuss here. However, there are certain analogies that can be drawn. The self is to a great extent determined and formed by our surroundings, including interactions with others, others' perception of us and treatment of us, and circumstances in our environment. When there is a sudden change in the surroundings, the self is bound to be affected. In other words, what feels like travel to an alternate universe changes the self. I no longer fully know who I am, or what I am like, because the old reference points have shifted. When I think about myself, I constantly need to consider the world in which I live as a point of comparison. It is thus impossible for me to stay just as I was. And so it is not only the self-perception and self-knowledge that are altered and upset, but also my sense of myself *as a self.* I not only lose my grip on who I am; who I am changes as well.

The analogy to the Twin Earth case consists in the change of reference points when we conceive of ourselves. Thus, when I move between worlds and think and speak of myself, I am referring to the old self that I left behind in the previous world, just like Oscar is still referring to H_2O even though he is pointing at what is actually XYZ after his arrival on Twin Earth. I will still be using some of the points of reference from the old world and refer to myself as I was back there. Perhaps this will change with time. As I grow into the new conditions in the new world, and into this new self of mine, I may come to refer to the new self when speaking of myself, using new points of reference. But this may be something we cannot know yet.

EXTENDED MIND

Another aspect of how our mental life relies on our environment can be explained through the so-called extended mind thesis. According to this theory, originally presented in 1998 by Andy Clark and David Chalmers,[4] our mental states do not only take place inside our heads or even inside our bodies, but extend to our surroundings. We form our surroundings and adjust them to our needs in order to aid our thinking. Some obvious examples are our use of writing instruments, whether they are a pen and paper, a typewriter, or a computer, that help us not only get our thoughts across to others but even to form them and develop. Clark and Chalmers describe a fictional Alzheimer's patient, Otto, who is going to the Museum of Modern Art on 53rd Street in New York. As Otto suffers from memory loss, he carries a notebook where he has written down his directions for how to get there. The notebook serves as a source of Otto's memory. Other examples of an extended mind can include various objects in our homes and workplaces that we place in ways that make our mental activities easier. It can be of great significance to place things such that they can be conveniently reached for the performance of various activities we consider important, whether they concern our emotional life, communication, forming of opinions, or fulfilling our duties and commitments.

Thus, the placement of things in our near environment can have a great effect on what and how we think and perform. If I need to spend hours looking for a writing instrument, I am not writing in the meantime, and if there is much distraction around me, I cannot focus on doing what I had intended to do. When circumstances change, such as during a move, this system is disturbed. Most people know how it can take some time to get settled in a new place, getting into a daily routine that makes it possible to focus and get things done. It has been pointed out how important it is to have a safe home for these purposes, as without a safe home, various things that others find easy will require considerably more effort.[5]

After a move to an alternate universe, this system is disturbed. Most of us are at home and in that sense in a familiar setting, so we do not have to spend time remembering where we keep our house keys or figuring out the best use of storage space for our pots and pans. But many of us are using our homes in very different ways from before, with the addition of great stress. In this way, our homes are made unfamiliar and our surroundings are made unfamiliar—and challenging. And we now have to learn how to navigate this new world—to discover a new country that seems to be located in the footprint of the old.

INDIVIDUALISTIC AND SOCIAL SELF

What I have been describing are things that can have a significant effect on a person's self-conception. For example, forming a number of new opinions on things one has not considered before is bound to affect one's self-image. Our opinions on various things are an important aspect of who we are, or who we think we are. Thus, our self-knowledge will be impacted and our self-image will be altered. We see and hear people having strong opinions on various things regarding the plague and we feel compelled to respond: Am I for or against face mask use? Am I happy with the various actions taken by my authorities? Do I think more should be done in response to this unprecedented situation, or perhaps less? How long do I expect these unusual circumstances to last? Will this be over in a month? Six months? A year, or perhaps several years? On what can I build my stance? What information can I trust?

While our self-conception may to some extent seem individualistic (Who am I? What are my opinions?), the self is also to a great extent social and relational, contingent on interactions with and perceptions by others, on relationships, and so forth. This social aspect of the self is, if anything, more affected than the individualistic aspect by our move to an alternate universe. So much has changed when it comes to interactions and relationships. Physical proximity and touch have been reduced and norms for civility in social interactions have changed. Handshakes are an obvious example: While it would previously be considered rude under various circumstances to forgo a handshake, it is now rude and inconsiderate to insist upon a handshake or even just to offer one. Many of us have also been self-isolating, either due to regulations set by authorities or on our own initiative, so suggesting a meeting in person may now be considered too forward or pushy. Less time spent in the vicinity of friends, family members, colleagues or random people in public spaces has resulted in feelings of loneliness and an increased sense of social awkwardness for many. Others had to spend great amounts of time within the walls of their homes with their same family members for extended periods of time, putting added strain on relationships.

All this has repercussions for the social self. We may suddenly find ourselves on opposite sides of a heated debate with people we previously were aligned with, and even experience hostility from them. On the other hand, we may find ourselves in unison with unexpected strangers, even on the other side of the world, joined in collective defense against the pandemic.

THE MORAL SELF

The whole world changed almost overnight, and great numbers of people have endured loss of employment and grief over loved ones, and had to rearrange their lives completely with enormous inconvenience and even hardship. Understandably, people are frustrated and angry and may feel a need to direct their frustrations at individuals or groups as morally blameworthy. Fighting a common enemy can sometimes have the effect of uniting people; they will work together, united against an outside threat. In this particular case, the "enemy" is not a thinking being who can be the target of blame in any moral sense. Thus, people may instead begin to turn against one another or try to locate someone at whom they can direct their anger. This pandemic has shifted us back and forth between feeling united, or "all in this together," as we react against a nonhuman entity, and turning against one another as we look for sources of bad decisions and badly executed actions, compete for medical resources and vaccines, and search for a target of our anger and fear.

In addition to this, we have come to fear one another and to be feared by others. We worry about transmission of the disease from others; we worry that our loved ones will become infected. We may also worry about becoming vectors ourselves and transmitting the virus to someone at risk. Some of us may experience fear when we pass others in the street—or just feel intense anxiety when encountering other people in general. This might be magnified if the "other" somehow differs from our own social circle or belongs to a lower social class.[6]

Public discourse can narrate, and thus reify, certain groups as threatening. In the United States, given months of racist official rhetoric, this has taken the form of prejudice against any Asian-appearing individuals. Another example involves international travelers in Iceland. That country is an island with only 340,000 inhabitants, and for many people, it seemed like a worthy goal to keep it more or less free of the COVID-19 virus in order to be able to minimize social distancing regulations, allowing the inhabitants to live freely without worrying about infection risk. In order to achieve this, heavy restrictions at the borders were necessary, including mandatory testing and a five-day quarantine for everyone entering. But in the first half of 2021, news began to appear of incoming travelers skipping their mandated five-day quarantine. Heated discussions ensued about possible ways to prevent this, and hostility toward anyone traveling to the country from abroad grew among the public. People entering the country came to be called "travel junkies," accused of being oblivious to their privilege and careless about spreading a lethal disease—if not downright amoral. International travelers are, of course, a very diverse group, and people travel for a number of reasons, including pressing personal ones. A significant proportion of travelers to and from Iceland during the pandemic included Eastern European workers residing in Iceland and working in low-income jobs; hardly what one would normally identify as a privileged group in comparison to the "locals." And needless to say, a great majority of travelers did follow the quarantine mandate meticulously. News began to emerge of people being accosted and verbally abused in public places because they had a suntan and thus looked as if they might have just arrived from some sunnier place abroad.[7]

Hostility toward international travelers is most likely a temporary phenomenon, especially since people who happen to have traveled during the pandemic are not readily identifiable as a social group for the long term, and there is not a strong historical or cultural predisposition for hostility toward people traveling for different reasons. Hostility toward ethnic and racial groups in connection with the pandemic is much more worrisome in that respect. But both are examples of how easily people can come to make new distinctions between in-groups and out-groups. Furthermore, the animosity toward people entering from abroad seems strongly connected to the tendency to think of danger as coming from the outside.

With increased surveillance, attitudes toward authority have changed considerably. In many countries all over the world, citizens have to submit to various checkups, answer questions about where they are going and why, get special permission for travel, and even have surveillance apps on their smartphones.[8] While these actions may be necessary in response to the pandemic, they clearly involve privacy infringements and limitations of individual freedom that most of us are not accustomed to and that would have seemed unthinkable not very long ago. Thus, people's relationship to strangers and authorities is bound to change.

What I have described here involves changes, often radical, in our moral selves—changes at the core of who we are. As a result of the pandemic, we have quickly been forced to adapt our moral views to the circumstances. We have had to take a stance not only on various social-distancing norms, mask wearing, and so on, but also on what kinds of behavior we consider responsible or irresponsible in light of the pandemic. We have taken up various moral views on things we had never considered before, or at least not in this particular light. As a result, each of us now holds strong moral opinions that we did not have before and that may even seem contrary to our previous moral views. We are even angered when we encounter behavior that conflicts with those views. In the most extreme cases, people have expressed hostility toward others and demanded strict regulations of behavior, increased surveillance of people's daily lives, and heavy enforcement of those regulations. While strict regulations and surveillance may in some cases be necessary under the current circumstances, these views are new for many of us, as are the strong moral feelings that often accompany them.

WORK

In his 1932 essay "In Praise of Idleness,"[9] Bertrand Russell argued for a shorter workday for everyone. A part of his argument was that with more time for leisure, people would be more likely to create works of art and have fruitful thoughts and discussions; in other words, our cultural life would flourish. This may suggest that there is an important aspect of the self, the creative and freely thinking self, that may have more opportunity to thrive when we are free from the duties and restrictions created by formal employment. Under current pandemic circumstances, workload and opportunities for leisure may have become more unevenly distributed than before. While some people have had more free time, whether due to unemployment or because they have saved the time otherwise spent commuting to and from work, others have experienced a heavier workload than usual. However, there are reasons to think that many of us have at least begun to reflect more on the role of work in our lives and its effects on our self-perception.[10]

In our modern Western society, most of us have been accustomed to defining people in terms of their professional training and activity. In many ways, that is to be expected. What a person spends most of their days doing or thinking about is likely to be a significant factor in who they are and what they are like. But, especially now, many of us have been going beyond that in our dedication to our work and workplace, and we fully define ourselves in terms of our profession. I have sometimes wondered what it would be like to suddenly be on another planet, or in another world, where the professional environment to which I have gotten accustomed did not exist. What would I spend my days doing? What would others around me be doing? Would we have to redefine ourselves and others? As large numbers of people have lost their sources of employment and many others have experienced great changes in their working arrangements and have worked from home, our previous ways of thinking about this have become unsettled. Some of us have begun to reflect on and question the importance of working life for one's identity. Of course, those who have lost their source of income due to loss of employment may feel that they do not have the same luxury in their reflection as those who have secure employment. Being able to get by and make ends meet is crucial. However, both loss of employment and altered arrangements at work may prompt people to reflect more on themselves as working people and on the importance of their identification with a certain profession or a dedication to a workplace. How important is this particular job to me? Would I still feel like "me" if I were to have a different type of job, or no job?

CONCLUSION

I have pointed out various ways in which the self is strongly affected by the move between universes resulting from the COVID-19 pandemic. These effects may, of course, differ greatly depending on people's varied circumstances. Also, as I write this, the pandemic has by no means ended, even though vaccinations have begun and people are beginning to catch glimpses of the light at the end of the tunnel. We still do not know how long the tunnel is or what exactly will greet us at the end.

What I can tell you is this: When you move to an alternate universe, you can expect to be changed. Expect the length of your residence there to be unpredictable. Expect to become confused, as time passes, about whether the alternate universe has become your permanent one. Expect to be unable to predict the nature of the universe that is to be your next stop. Expect the unexpected.

BIBLIOGRAPHY

Clark, Andy, and David Chalmers. "The Extended Mind." *Analysis* 58, no. 1 (1998): 7–19.

Couch, Danielle L., Priscilla Robinson, and Paul A. Komesaroff. "COVID-19—Extending Surveillance and the Panopticon." *Journal of Bioethical Inquiry* 17, no. 4 (2020): 809–14. https://doi.org/10.1007/s11673-020-10036-5.

Lingis, Alphonso. "The New Fear of One Another." *Journal of Bioethical Inquiry* 17, no. 4 (2020): 471–72. https://doi.org/10.1007/s11673-020-10035-6.

Nine, Cara. "The Wrong of Displacement: The Home as Extended Mind." *Journal of Political Philosophy* 26, no. 2 (2017): 240–57. https://doi.org/10.1111/jopp.12133.

O'Connor, Brian. *Idleness: A Philosophical Essay*. Princeton, NJ: Princeton University Press, 2018.

Pétursdóttir, Ása Ninna. "Sökuð um brot á sóttkví eftir að hafa tekið lit í íslenskri sól." Visir.is, 8 April 2021. https://www.visir.is/g/20212094623d/sokud-um-brot-a-sottkvi-eftir-ad-hafa-tekid-lit-i-islenskri-sol.

Putnam, Hilary. "Meaning and Reference." *Journal of Philosophy* 70, no. 19 (1973): 699–711. https://doi.org/10.2307/2025079.

Putnam, Hilary. “The Meaning of ‘Meaning,’” 215–711. In *Mind, Language, and Reality*. New York: Cambridge University Press, 1975.

Russell, Bertrand. “In Praise of Idleness.” In *In Praise of Idleness and Other Essays*. London: Unwin Books, 1973.

NOTES

1. Hilary Putnam, “Meaning and Reference,” *Journal of Philosophy* 70, no. 19 (1973).

2. Hilary Putnam, “The Meaning of ‘Meaning,’,” in *Mind, Language, and Reality* (New York: Cambridge University Press, 1975).

3. It is a part of the story that Oscar is living in a time before the molecular structure of water was discovered as H_2O, so he has no conception of H_2O as such.

4. Andy Clark and David Chalmers, “The Extended Mind,” *Analysis* 58, no. 1 (1998).

5. For an interesting discussion of this, including the effect of lack of a safe home on refugees, see Cara Nine, “The Wrong of Displacement,” *Journal of Political Philosophy* 26, no. 2 (2017), https://doi.org/10.1111/jopp.12133.

6. Alphonso Lingis, “The New Fear of One Another,” *Journal of Bioethical Inquiry* 17, no. 4 (2020), https://doi.org/10.1007/s11673-020-10035-6.

7. Ása Ninna Pétursdóttir, “Sökuð um brot á sóttkví eftir að hafa tekið lit í íslenskri sól,” Visir.is, April 8, 2021, https://www.visir.is/g/20212094623d/sokud-um-brot-a-sottkvi-eftir-ad-hafa-tekid-lit-i-islenskri-sol.

8. Danielle Couch, Priscilla Robinson, and Paul A. Komesaroff, “COVID-19—Extending Surveillance and the Panopticon,” *Journal of Bioethical Inquiry* 17, no. 4 (2020), https://doi.org/10.1007/s11673-020-10036-5.

9. Bertrand Russell, “In Praise of Idleness,” in *In Praise of Idleness and Other Essays* (London: Unwin Books, 1973).

10. Brian O’Connor criticizes various philosophical arguments condemning idleness in Brian O‘Connor, *Idleness: a Philosophical Essay* (Princeton, NJ: Princeton University Press, 2018).

Chapter 13

Viral Hope: When Quarantine Comes Home

Daniel Conway

Long before I was made aware of the COVID-19 virus, I decided to ask my undergraduate students to read *The Plague* (*La peste*; 1947) by Albert Camus. I also scheduled this reading assignment for the end of the spring 2020 semester, which, as it turns out, meant the students would be reading and thinking about the quarantine of Oran while enduring their very own quarantine in Texas.[1]

FATHER PANELOUX

The central figure of acknowledged religious authority in *The Plague* is Father Paneloux, a Jesuit priest who ministers to the Catholic faithful of Oran. When the plague strikes, the "ecclesiastical authorities" in Oran commence a "Week of Prayer," which culminates in a High Mass on the feast day of St. Roch.[2] Intending to account for the provenance and possible remission of the plague, Father Paneloux takes to his pulpit to deliver the sermon. He explains the outbreak of plague as the consequence of God having "turned His face away from us," which he interprets (and promptly justifies) as a proportional response to their persistent habit of taking His "divine mercy" for granted.[3] As Paneloux develops this account of the plague, he neither minces his words nor spares the feelings of his parishioners:

> If today the plague is in your midst, that is because the hour has struck for taking thought. The just man need have no fear, but the evildoer has good cause to tremble. For plague is the flail of God and the world His threshing-floor, and implacably He will thresh out His harvest until the wheat is separated from the

chaff. There will be more chaff than wheat, few chosen of the many called. Yet this calamity was not willed by God.[4]

On the face of it, there is nothing particularly remarkable or unique about this sermon. Priests and other religious leaders regularly attribute natural disasters and outbreaks of disease to the upsurge or persistence of sin (or similar lapses, whether real or perceived). When Hurricane Katrina swamped the city of New Orleans, for example, various celebrity preachers blamed the devastation on what they viewed as the city's permissive tolerance of homosexuality.

In making this particular appeal, however, Father Paneloux commits what will later be revealed to be a tactical rhetorical misstep, from which he will adroitly—if chillingly—recover in a second sermon. In this first sermon, his parishioners are assured that the just among them "need have no fear," which implies that the plague has been engineered to target only the unjust—the proverbial "chaff"—in their midst. Lest they surmise that their God is either inexpert or inattentive or whimsical as a harvester of souls, the just among those assembled for Paneloux's sermon may go about their business as usual. According to Father Paneloux, in fact, the plague is an undeserved gift from God—and, so, evidence of His love—albeit in the form of a stern admonition to return to the path of righteousness. As Paneloux explains, God has unleashed the plague as a means of claiming the full attention of the distracted faithful: "Now, at last, you know the hour has struck to bend your thoughts to first and last things."[5]

For some, of course, the effort involved in "bending" their thoughts will be to no avail. If "many are called" to the threshing floor, the odds of any individual finding himself among the "wheat" of the accursed city are prohibitively long. And although it is potentially comforting to the *über*-righteous that "the just man need have no fear," the plague itself displays no corresponding deference. As the inexorable epidemiology of the plague dictates, the just and the unjust of Oran should expect to be stricken (or not) indiscriminately, owing more to considerations of luck than of character. Even if the "just" find themselves spared, moreover, their children, friends, and neighbors will not be so fortunate. In claiming the plague as a vector of "divine mercy," Paneloux risks projecting his God as either cruel or inept. In any event, his first sermon has encouraged his parishioners to orient themselves to the future either by way of false hope (the "just") or by way of unwarranted desperation (the "unjust"). Hence the need, as we shall see, for the corrective provided by the approach he takes in his second sermon.

Although Father Paneloux is a Jesuit priest—that is, an ordained member of the Society of Jesus—his preferred interpretation of the plague confirms his allegiance to a different, far older source of moral authority. (Whether this allegiance is situational and new, planted in him by the escalation of the pandemic, is difficult to know. What seems clear is that he is not exactly reluctant to defend the biblical justice to which he now bears eloquent witness.) Whereas Jesus appears in the New Testament as generally merciful, eager to forgive the trespasses of nearly everyone He encounters, including many of those who have wronged Him, Paneloux invokes the wrath of an angry deity determined to enforce an archaic canon of retributive justice. Paneloux's God, who dials up a devastating plague to claim the attention of those mortals whom He loves, is more at home in what Christians prefer to call the Old Testament. Channeling the (doom) prophets of the Hebrew Bible, Paneloux endeavors to heap blame (and responsibility) for the plague on those preoccupied parishioners whose lapses have persisted for far too long:

> And this is why, wearied of waiting for you to come to Him, He loosed on you this visitation: as He has visited all the cities that offended against Him since the dawn of history. Now you are learning your lesson, the lesson that was learned by Cain and his offspring, by the people of Sodom and Gomorrah, by Job and Pharaoh, by all that hardened their hearts against Him.[6]

Cain and his East-of-Eden offspring? Sodom and Gomorrah? Pharaoh? Does Paneloux seriously mean to suggest that the plague is evidence of the biblical-grade evil proliferating unchecked in Oran? Here we might note that whatever the evil in question is believed to entail, it is nowhere considered to involve the injustice encoded in the ongoing colonial presence of the French—and of the Catholicism they have imported—in a commercially strategic port city in North Africa.

After delivering his memorable sermon, Father Paneloux is persuaded to join the recently assembled sanitary brigades, which, under the leadership of Jean Tarrou, are tasked with restoring sanitary conditions, limiting the spread of the contagion, tending to victims of the plague, and organizing the collection of sick, feverish, and dead bodies. Heedlessly placing themselves at the epicenter of the plague, (most of) the members of the sanitary brigades find meaning, purpose, and fellowship amid the stench and decay of the quarantined city. Despite—or, rather, because of—the proximity of death and the high probability of contagion, they learn to treasure their hours together and create for themselves an intensity of quotidian meaning that previously had been missing from their lives. Their work is routine, filthy, humbling, and eminently dangerous, yet it suits them well.

In keeping with his Jesuit training and vocation, Father Paneloux pitches in and becomes a regular contributor to the work of the sanitary brigades. Although he continues to insist that the citizens of Oran have brought the plague on themselves, he nevertheless affirms the mission of tending to the afflicted. He thus strikes a familiar balance between blaming the victims of the plague and assisting them and their loved ones in their hours of need. In doing so, moreover, he confirms his dual allegiance to the wrathful God of the Hebrew prophets and the merciful God of the New Testament. An unexamined irony of this dual allegiance is that Paneloux's support of the sanitary brigades actually may serve to protect or even resuscitate some of those whose neglect of their God has brought the plague to their city. If some of these scofflaws are also members of Paneloux's own parish, moreover, he may find himself in an unanticipated bind of double jeopardy: Having failed in his spiritual ministry while succeeding in his secular ministry, *he* may be responsible for prolonging the duration of the plague.

ALL OR NOTHING

This delicate balance is challenged soon enough by a grave turn of events. A young boy, Philippe Othon, son of the local magistrate, has been stricken by the plague. Can it be said that this child, innocent by all accounts, deserves the plague as a punishment for his sins? Even if one were inclined to classify the youngster as collateral damage in a larger exercise of divine retribution, one would be hard pressed to see (much less defend) the justice and mercy of the deity whose will ordains the suffering of blameless children. Here Camus lends his authorial voice to a chorus raised by some of the leading European critics of Christianity, including Voltaire, Fyodor Dostoevsky, and Friedrich Nietzsche: How can a just deity allow for the suffering of innocent children? How can anyone continue to speak of a divine plan, even if hidden from our view, that eventually will deliver us unto the best of all possible worlds? And how can anyone find love and mercy in a warning shot that takes the life of an innocent child?

And the situation worsens. Young Othon has been injected with an experimental serum that is meant to relieve some of the most severe of the symptoms associated with the plague. The hope attached to his recovery is thus suggestive of the larger (and equally desperate) hope for a more expansive, citywide victory over the plague and its carriers. But the serum does not work as planned, and young Othon's condition continues to deteriorate. He is clearly deathbound. The serum also has the unwanted side effect of causing him to endure violent spasms and wracking convulsions. If anything, the serum exacerbates his suffering. What deity has authorized this ordeal?

Following the death of young Othon, witnessed in person by Father Paneloux, the Jesuit faces what for others might have qualified as a crisis of faith. The deceased was hardly a sinner of note, yet he was claimed by the plague, which Paneloux has publicly identified as the "flail" of his God. At least with respect to the work of the sanitary brigades, moreover, the citizens of Oran had recently rededicated themselves to a life of selfless, Christlike service, which, one might have thought, could have allayed the wrath of their displeased God. Yet the child perished nonetheless, while enduring an excruciatingly painful death.

To his credit, Father Paneloux faces up to the ensuing challenge to his faith (and, so, to his religious authority). Rather than question his God or subject his faith to reexamination, however, Paneloux doubles down on his earlier attempt at theodicy, urging the faithful of Oran to do likewise. In a second sermon, he dramatically raises the stakes of his exhortation to his parishioners: "My brothers, a time of testing has come for us all. We must believe everything or deny everything. And who among you, I ask, would dare to deny everything?"[7]

If the death of the innocent child is incident to God's will, the priest advises, then it must become incident to the will of all those who wish to remain among God's faithful.[8] The narrator of the novel, whom we eventually learn to be none other than Dr. Rieux, refers to this appeal as obliging the faithful to "acquire and practice the greatest of all virtues: that of the All or Nothing."[9] What Rieux has in mind here is a rhetorical ploy that becomes both effective and necessary in times of unprecedented uncertainty: To cast doubt on the wisdom of God's plan, simply because a seemingly blameless child has perished of the plague, is to cast doubt on everything one has thus far taken to be true, good, and just. Lest they find themselves morally and spiritually adrift in a godless cosmos, Paneloux's parishioners would do well to follow his lead and immediately accommodate themselves to the inscrutable justice of their God.

Rather than question the justice and mercy of his God, Father Paneloux questions the (relative) value he and others have attached to the life of an innocent child. In effect, his second sermon transforms the boy into a convenient scapegoat whose painful, seemingly pointless death allows—and perhaps compels—the faithful of Oran to align their will with the "All-or-Nothing" mandate of Paneloux's God. Rather than "dare to deny everything," *à la* Ivan Karamazov, they resolve to "believe everything"—including, apparently, what the author and narrator of *The Plague* both find to be incomprehensible. In so resolving, the priest implies, they will pass the test set before them. The death of the young boy is their God's gift to them.

According to the logic of Paneloux's second sermon, the death of the innocent boy proves that the citizens of Oran have not yet responded as needed to the warning the plague is supposed to have sounded. Just as they brought the plague upon themselves, as Paneloux confirmed in his first sermon, so they have now obliged their God to take the life of the innocent child. Having ignored (or not taken seriously enough) the original warning shot, they have compelled their otherwise merciful God to issue an even sterner warning. The death of young Othon is thus presented (and affirmed) as the event that will (finally) claim the attention of the distracted faithful and thereby turn back the plague. Here we should take note of a significant escalation in the rhetoric employed by Father Paneloux. In his first sermon, as we know, he was careful to insist that the plague was *not* the will of their God. In his second sermon, however, he confirms that the death of young Othon is not only the will of their God but also the will of those who wish to withstand the test to which they have been subjected.

For some, to be sure, the faith expressed by Father Paneloux is a bridge too far, while for others it is a bridge to nowhere. Still others will find strength or stability in the bracing, either/or clarity of the position he has staked out. For his own part, Camus endeavors to reveal the madness that is encoded in the horrifyingly rational calculus that Father Paneloux invites his parishioners to adopt. His point in revealing this madness is to demonstrate that the hope arising from Paneloux's faith, a hope linked to a divine plan that authorizes the suffering and death of innocent children, is even more lethal than the plague itself. The lesson learned by the other members of the sanitary brigades, who take it upon themselves to create meaning in *this* moment, the only moment granted to them, is lost on Father Paneloux.

STUDENT RESPONSES TO *THE PLAGUE*

In my undergraduate courses and modules in philosophy of religion, I typically spend quite a bit of time discussing the various theodicies of influence in the Western (or European) traditions of philosophy and theology. In furthering this pedagogical objective, I often invite the students to read *The Plague* and evaluate the wisdom of Father Paneloux's quarantine-prompted sermons. This past year was different because we were contemplating the quarantine of Oran while complying in real time with quarantine measures imposed upon us under the plaguelike conditions of the COVID-19 pandemic. As a result, the questions I raised with my students were not received as abstract, academic, or hypothetical, and they were not restricted to the imagined confines of a relatively obscure colonial port city on the northern coast of Algeria.

Owing to their own experience of the pandemic, my quarantined students were unusually attentive to the rhetorical power of Father Paneloux's sermons. As they had come to know from their own experience, conditions of plague and quarantine intensify the desire for answers and amplify the need for meaning. Like Paneloux's plague-wary parishioners, my students understood themselves to be a captive audience. They furthermore understood that captivity breeds uncertainty and desperation, which can lead those who are quarantined to take seriously explanations that under normal conditions would hold no appeal. Even those students who disagreed with Father Paneloux, including those who deemed him evil, cold, or heartless, were able to appreciate (and respond to) the power of his rhetorical appeals.

What Father Paneloux senses or intuits, they realized, is that in times of crisis and uncertainty, people need to be united; the world they face together must make sense, even if the sense it makes is unflattering or daunting to outsiders and onlookers. Under such conditions, or so Father Paneloux understands, *any* explanation of the plague, including the victim-blaming explanation he serves up, is preferable to no explanation at all. If no other or better explanations are available, as we have seen, a scapegoat must be identified—*not* because the scapegoat in question is demonstrably guilty, but because the stability of the society or polity hangs in the balance.

This time around, in other words, my students were able to appreciate that Father Paneloux's sermons, even if considered spiteful, served a purpose. They recognized in themselves a desire for meaning, for explanation, and for a second (or third) chance to hew to the path of righteousness. Indeed, what is the alternative? To concede that the plague comes and goes for no reason at all, that its periodic resurgence is a permanent feature of our unguarded world? That our best efforts will secure at most a temporary respite? That no deity hears—much less heeds—our petitionary prayers?

These alternatives, of course, are precisely what Camus means to recommend to his target readership. The absurdity of the human condition is revealed, he believes, in the collision of our natural desire for permanent meaning with the brute intransigence of the natural world/godless cosmos we inhabit.[10] According to Camus, we never will achieve the validation we understandably seek, owing not to any sin or lapse on our part, original or otherwise, but to the nature and the structure of the world in which we find ourselves. At the same time, however, we are free to create transient and limited meaning through our choices, that is, our acts of "rebellion" against the absurdity of our situation.[11]

The centerpiece example of such acts of "rebellion" is the uncompelled work of the sanitary brigades, especially as this work is organized and conducted by Jean Tarrou, the hero of the novel. Despite not believing in God, Tarrou is determined to become a "saint,"[12] which is why he insists on placing himself at the epicenter of the plague. If the "good man" is he "who infects hardly anyone," as Tarrou insists to Rieux, then "the saint" Tarrou has in mind must be one who *also* assists those who are afflicted, even if doing so places him in peril.[13] And, as we know, Tarrou succumbs to the plague, which may mean that he achieved in death the goal he had set for himself. Tarrou's death wish, expressed in his zeal to immerse himself in the work of the sanitary brigades, thus reveals an underlying life wish, wherein the quality of the life he chose for himself trumped the more familiar desire to extend indefinitely the duration of one's life.

CONCLUSION

I will close this reflection with three observations:

First, drawing on their unique, first-person experience of the COVID-19 pandemic, my quarantined students exhibited a keen appreciation of the role of religious figures and religious authorities in stabilizing a society or polity rocked by uncertainty. They became acutely aware that Father Paneloux's sermons were meant to succeed as secular interventions, independent of their merit as spiritual or theological interventions. This was the case, or so I surmise, because the very questions raised and answered by Paneloux's sermons were raised (and occasionally answered) by my students, their friends and family members, and their various comrades in quarantine. For the first time in my teaching career, the social and psychological costs of quarantine were known (and not merely imagined) by my students.

Second, alert to the rhetorical effect *on them* of Father Paneloux's sermons, my quarantined students were unusually adventurous in considering the merit of Camus's opposition to hope. Typically, in a class like this one, Camus does not receive a sympathetic hearing. In the past, his opposition to hope and his relentless attention to the meaningfulness of the present moment have struck my students as both extreme and unviable. They have been reluctant to give up their hopes for the future, in large part because doing so strikes them as alien to the human condition as they know it.

My quarantined students were similarly reluctant to give up their hopes for the future, but they were significantly more sympathetic to the imperative, especially as it is dramatized in the work of the sanitary brigades, to create meaning for themselves in the here and now.[14] Even if they were not willing to live a hope-less existence, they understood that some expressions of hope, most notably those authorized by standard theodicies, can be as devastating in their own right as the onset of plague.

The recognition achieved on this occasion by my students was most evident in their commendably intrepid efforts to distinguish meaningfully between those species of hope that *improve* the quality of life and those that *detract* from the quality of life. Following the lead of Camus, they were able to appreciate that what we might call "blind" hope is at best a product of a self-protective impulse or mechanism. Under the impress of "blind" hope, they realized, they were likely to remain locked in a posture of childlike naivete and vulnerability, hoping for a "best" that was not likely ever to materialize. Taking their cues from Tarrou (and perhaps Rieux), my students realized that an informed, adult expression of hope would allow them to reap the full measure of the meaning and value that are in fact available to them. This particular insight was especially resonant with those students who understood themselves to be committed by their moral and religious training to bring about the better world their hopes had disclosed to them.

Third, my quarantined students were noticeably more alert to the (admittedly counterintuitive) suggestion that an aspiration to "sainthood" is possible even for those who do not believe in God. As we know, this unusual articulation of religiosity is advanced in *The Plague* by the novel's hero, Jean Tarrou, who not only organizes the sanitary brigades but also works tirelessly to care for the afflicted. Indeed, my quarantined students were surprisingly (and refreshingly) receptive to Tarrou's rebellious aspiration to "sainthood," which he defines, privatively, in terms of limiting the damage one does to others. By way of honoring my quarantine-bound students, I yield my final words to Tarrou, as he reveals to his friend, Rieux, the secret of a well-wrought life:

> The good man, the man who infects hardly anyone, is the man who has the fewest lapses of attention. And it needs tremendous will-power, a never ending tension of the mind, to avoid such lapses. Yes, Rieux, it's a wearying business, being plague-stricken. But it's still more wearying to refuse to be it.[15]

BIBLIOGRAPHY

Aronson, Ronald. "Albert Camus." In *The Stanford Encyclopedia of Philosophy*, Summer 2017, edited by Edward N. Zalta https://plato.stanford.edu/archives/sum2017/entries/camus/.

Camus, Albert. *The Plague*. Translated by Stuart Gilbert. New York: Random House/Vintage International, 1991.

———. *The Rebel*. Translated by Anthony Bower. New York: Random House/Vintage International, 1991.

Zaretsky, Robert D. *Camus: Elements of a Life*. Ithaca, NY: Cornell University Press, 2010.

NOTES

1. An earlier version of this essay was published as D. Conway, (2020) "Faith under Quarantine: Lessons from Camus," 39–41, in *Religion in Quarantine: The Future of Religion in a Post-Pandemic World*, ed. H. Campbell (College Station, TX: Digital Religion Productions, 2020),https://doi.org/10.21423/religioninquarantine. I am grateful to Anna Gotlib for her instructive comments on earlier drafts of this essay.

2. Albert Camus, *The Plague*, trans. Stuart Gilbert (New York: Random House/Vintage International, 1991), 92.
3. Camus, *The Plague*, 96.
4. Camus, *The Plague*, 95.
5. Camus, *The Plague*, 97.
6. Camus, *The Plague*, 97.
7. Camus, *The Plague*, 224.
8. Camus, *The Plague*, 225.
9. Camus, *The Plague*, 225.
10. Ronald Aronson, "Albert Camus," in *The Stanford Encyclopedia of Philosophy*, summer 2017, ed. Edward N. Zalta, section 3, https://plato.stanford.edu/archives/sum2017/entries/camus/.
11. I am indebted here to Aronson, "Albert Camus," sections 3.4–3.5; and Robert D. Zaretsky, *Camus: Elements of a Life* (Ithaca, NY: Cornell University Press, 2010), 107–10.
12. Camus, *The Plague*, 255.
13. Camus, *The Plague*, 253.
14. See Zaretsky, *Camus*, 85–89.
15. Camus, *The Plague*, 253.

Index

Italicized page numbers indicate illustrations.

About the Contributors

Alexios Alexander is assistant professor of political science at Eastern University, where he serves as program director for political science. His research and teaching focus on the history of political theory, philosophy of law, philosophy of language, and American political thought.

Joseph S. Biehl is the founder and executive director of the Gotham Philosophical Society. He holds a BA in philosophy from St. John's University and a PhD from the Graduate School and University Center, CUNY, and has taught philosophy for over twenty years. He is the coeditor (with Sharon Meagher and Samantha Noll) of *The Routledge Handbook of Philosophy of the City* (Routledge, 2019). He is currently writing *The Dawning of the Age of Protagoras*, a book on the perils and possibilities of living in a post-truth world.

Eyja M. Brynjarsdóttir is professor of philosophy at the University of Iceland. She has a PhD in philosophy from Cornell University (2007). Brynjarsdóttir often works on moral and other philosophical aspects of current events, most recently the COVID-19 pandemic and the #MeToo movement, and is interested in various issues within social philosophy, feminist philosophy, and applied ethics. Her publications include the monograph *The Reality of Money* (Rowman and Littlefield, 2018).

Daniel Conway is professor of philosophy and humanities, affiliate professor of religious studies and film studies, and courtesy professor in the TAMU School of Law and the George Bush School of Government and Public Service at Texas A&M University. He has lectured and published widely on topics in post-Kantian European philosophy, political theory, philosophy of religion, philosophy and literature, philosophy and film, American philosophy, law and humanities, and genocide studies.

Barrett Emerick is an associate professor of philosophy at St. Mary's College of Maryland. He writes and teaches about normative ethics, moral psychology, and social justice. He recently published an article called "The Limits of the Rights to Free Thought and Expression" in the *Kennedy Institute of Ethics Journal*. He is currently coauthoring a monograph on moral solidarity, moral repair, and restorative justice.

Anna Gotlib is an associate professor of philosophy at Brooklyn College CUNY, specializing in feminist bioethics/medical ethics, moral psychology, and philosophy of law. She received her PhD in philosophy from Michigan State University and a JD from Cornell Law School. Anna coedits the *International Journal of Feminist Approaches to Bioethics*. Her work has appeared in the *Kennedy Institute of Ethics Journal*, *Journal of Bioethical Inquiry*, *Journal of Medical Humanities*, *Hypatia*, *Aeon/Psyche*, and other publications. She also edited two volumes on moral psychology for Rowman and Littlefield International—*The Moral Psychology of Sadness* (2017) and *The Moral Psychology of Regret* (2019). Currently, she is working on a monograph on identity, memory, and trauma, and in spring/summer of 2022 she was a Fulbright Specialist Scholar at the University of Iceland.

Ruth Groenhout is the distinguished professor of health care ethics at the University of North Carolina Charlotte. Her primary areas of research focus on healthcare ethics, feminist theory, and ethical theory. Her books include *Care Ethics and Social Structures in Medicine*, *Connected Lives: Human Nature and an Ethics of Care*, and *Philosophy, Feminism and Faith*, coedited with Marya Bower. Recent articles include "Reformed Theology and Conscientious Refusal of Medical Treatment" in *Christian Bioethics*, "Beauvoir and the Biological Body" in *The Blackwell Companion to Simone de Beauvoir*, "Of Medicine and Monsters: Rationing and an Ethics of Care" in *Care Ethics and Political Theory* and "Virtue and a Feminist Ethics of Care" in *Virtues and Their Vices*.

Claire Elise Katz is professor of philosophy at Texas A&M University. She is the author of *Levinas, Judaism, and the Feminine* (Indiana, 2003), *Levinas and the Crisis of Humanism* (Indiana, 2013), and *An Introduction to Modern Jewish Philosophy* (IB Tauris and Bloomsbury, 2014). She is the editor of *Growing up with Philosophy Camp* (Rowman and Littlefield, 2020), *Philosophy Camps for Youth* (Rowman and Littlefield, 2021), and, with Laura Trout, *Emmanuel Levinas: Critical Assessments* (Routledge, 2005).

Eva Feder Kittay is distinguished professor of philosophy at Stony Brook University/SUNY; a senior fellow of the Stony Brook Center for Medical Humanities, Compassionate Care and Bioethics; and an affiliate of the Women's Studies Program. She is the recipient of a Guggenheim Fellowship, an NEH Fellowship, and the APA and Phi Beta Kappa Lebowitz Prize. She has also been recognized for her work in feminist philosophy, being named Woman Philosopher of the Year (2003–2004) by the Society for Women in Philosophy and having chaired the Committee on the Status of Women (1997–2001). Her book *Love's Labor: Essays on Women, Equality, and Dependency* (Routledge, 1999) has received international attention and has been translated into Japanese and Italian. She has edited many journal issues in feminist philosophy and the philosophy of disability and has published more than eighty-five articles and book chapters.

Corey McCall taught philosophy at Elmira College in upstate New York for a number of years and he currently teaches for the Cornell Prison Education Program at Cornell University. His work focuses on ethical and aesthetic questions across Continental, American, and African philosophical traditions. His most recent book is the coedited collection *Decolonizing American Philosophy* (SUNY, 2021).

Jamie L. Nelson is professor emerita in Michigan State University's Philosophy Department. She works in philosophy of language and of literature and moral psychology, but the brunt of her publications focus on issues in bioethics; these include *The Patient in the Family*, with Hilde Lindemann (Routledge 2002); *Hippocrates's Maze* (Rowman and Littlefield 2002); and scores of articles and chapters. A book on the bioethics of transgender is currently in preparation.

Jennifer Scuro was visiting faculty in disability studies at Miami University in Ohio in 2021 before being appointed assistant professor in philosophy and ethics at Molloy College in New York. She is the author of *The Pregnancy ≠ Childbearing Project: A Phenomenology of Miscarriage* (Rowman and Littlefield International, 2017) and *Addressing Ableism: Philosophical Questions via Disability Studies* (Lexington Books, 2017). During the pandemic, she sculpted figures of women philosophers under the series title #IntellectualInheritance and worked on publishing in public philosophy, including a short series of YouTube videos, with philosophical counselor Monica Vilhauer, titled *Rogue Philosophers*. She is currently completing a certificate in trauma response and crisis intervention from Rutgers University and has begun working on a manuscript on the intersection of trauma and disability.

Kevin Timpe works in the philosophy department at Calvin University, where he currently holds the William H. Jellema Chair. Most of his scholarship focuses on the philosophy of disability, virtue ethics, the metaphysics of free will, and philosophy of religion. He is also the president of 22 Advocacy, a disability advocacy company that specializes in protecting disabled students in public education.

Vanessa Wills is a political philosopher, ethicist, educator, and activist working in Washington, DC. She is assistant professor of philosophy at the George Washington University. In 2019–2020, she was additionally the DAAD Visiting Chair in Ethics and Practice at Ludwig-Maximilian-Universität's Munich Center for Ethics. Her areas of specialization are moral, social, and political philosophy, nineteenth-century German philosophy (especially Karl Marx), and the philosophy of race. Her research is importantly informed by her study of Marx's work, and focuses on the ways in which economic and social arrangements can inhibit or promote the realization of values such as freedom, equality, and human development. She is on the editorial board of *Spectre Journal*, a biannual journal of Marxist theory, strategy, and analysis.

www.ingramcontent.com/pod-product-compliance
Ingram Content Group UK Ltd.
Pitfield, Milton Keynes, MK11 3LW, UK
UKHW041835031026
15587UKWH00002B/789

9 781538 154045